Praise for Terry and *50+ Natural Health Secrets Proven to Change Your Life!*

"Terry Lemerond is a maverick. He is a legend in his own time as it pertains to the field of evidence-based natural medicine. His passion for knowledge and his strong, heartfelt desire to share it has made the world a much better place. I am honored to not only know this man, but to have had the chance to work with him and learn from him."

—Holly Lucille, ND, RN, nationally recognized educator, practitioner, author, natural products consultant, and television and radio host

"Have you been failed by the medical profession? Help is on the way! After 40 years as a physician, and having reviewed tens of thousands of studies, I have found that there is a simple way to learn what natural treatments will be future superstars. Simply see what Terry Lemerond is talking about today!"

—Jacob Teitelbaum, MD, Director of the Fatigue and Fibromyalgia Practitioners Network, practitioner, researcher, and expert in chronic pain. Author of multiple best-selling books including *Fatigued to Fantastic*. Lead author of the SHINE protocol for Chronic Fatigue Syndrome and Fibromyalgia

"Terry Lemerond is a walking encyclopedia when it comes to natural cures, botanicals, and nutraceuticals. The formulator of over 400 products, he knows as much about what works and what doesn't as anyone I've ever met. He's one of a handful of people in the natural products industry who really deserves the designation 'icon.' I've learned a ton from Terry—read this book and you'll see why!"

—Jonny Bowden, PhD, CNS, best-selling author, radio host, speaker, and national media health expert on weight loss, nutrition, and health with six national certifications in personal training and exercise

"Terry has been a pioneer for natural health products for close to fifty years, and through these years he has found countless, life-changing ingredients that really have made a tremendous impact on people's health. I have never met anyone during my tenure in the natural health industry with such vision for finding the best quality and unique ingredients around the world. Not only has Terry contributed incredible products and been the first to introduce some of these ingredients to North America, he has inspired so many with his kindness, passion, dedication, and love for people and natural health. He speaks from a place of personal experience, and through this his love for what he does shines brightly. I am blessed to know Terry both personally and professionally, and it is an honor to call him my friend."

—Karlene Karst, RD, best-selling author, and recognized authority on the role of natural food and wholesome ingredients in nutrition, author, and founder of Sea-licious

"Due to my academic research, I have had the privilege of getting to meet some of the leading authorities in the world on the medicinal benefits of botanicals and phytochemicals. However, I must say Terry is, without a question, one of the most well-versed and knowledgeable individuals I have ever had the privilege and honor of getting to know. His breadth of understanding on a large number of plants and herbs amazes me, but what is more fascinating is his depth of scientific knowledge on these products—which is truly remarkable and exceptional. All of this is fueled by Terry's unparalleled passion for learning and educating consumers on the health benefits of nature's cures."

—**Ajay Goel, PhD**, Professor and the Director of Translational Genomics and Oncology, and the Director of the Center for Gastrointestinal Research at the Baylor Scott & White Research Institute, Baylor University Medical Center in Dallas, TX., member of American Cancer Association for Research and the American Gastroenterology Association, and one of the top scientists in the world investigating botanical interventions.

"From the viewpoint of an editor of scientific journals on phytomedicine and phytotherapy research, this guide for the novice consumer of dietary supplements is surprisingly different from many handbooks on herbal medicines. This book was written by a pioneer in natural health products, a walking encyclopedia, and a revolutionary thinker. I want to emphasize that this evidence based information is a summary of selected medicinal plants and supplements, covering all of the most essential health conditions that is valuable for a consumer. The consumer should read this book."

—**Alexander Panossian PhD, Dr.Sc.**, has advanced research degrees in bioorganic chemistry and specializes in the study of adaptogenic herbs. He has authored or co-authored over 170 scientific publications. Dr. Panossian is a past Editor-in-Chief of *Phytomedicine*.

"Terry Lemerond is the reason I was drawn into the world of natural health. His passion is contagious and his magnificent knowledge of natural supplements set me on the road to becoming an integrative medicine practitioner and professional lecturer. I am proud to call him my teacher, my mentor, and my friend. His book is a perfect doorway into the world of clinically validated, highly effective natural interventions for some of the most serious health problems facing people today. If you have health questions, your answers begin in this book."

—**Cheryl Myers, RN, BA**, is an integrative health care professional, research liaison, author, lecturer, and natural products expert. Her blogs and columns can be found in *Taste for Life, MindBodyGreen,* and *Vitamin Retailer*.

50+ NATURAL HEALTH SECRETS

Proven to Change Your Life!

TERRY LEMEROND

Host and Publisher of Terry Talks Nutrition

WEBSITE, NEWSLETTER, AND INTERNET RADIO SHOW

Published by:

Terry Talks Nutrition

TerryTalksNutrition.com

ISBN: 978-1-7321959-0-5

Editor: Cheryl Myers
Cover: Jill Baker
Writers: Julie Hoerth, Lexi Loch, Michele Olson, Dan Stearns
Interior: Gary A. Rosenberg • www.thebookcouple.com

Printed in the United States of America

10   9   8   7   6   5   4   3   2   1

Contents

Foreword

by Dr. Benny Antony

Dr. Benny Antony has a doctorate in organic chemistry. He was instrumental in establishing Arjuna Natural Extracts Ltd., a pioneering company in the field of herbal and spice extracts, where he serves as founder and director. With 27 years of experience, he is considered a leading expert in the field. Under his guidance, more than 45 best selling herbal extracts have been developed. He is credited with 28 patents, over 35 pending patent applications, 17 publications, and several awards of recognition in his field of research.

• •

About Terry

I am delighted to write about Terry Lemerond because of my tremendous respect and admiration for him. I learned from him that a man is what he believes. And the greatest power in the universe resides within oneself. Terry believes that it is the power of the mind that makes one good, bad, sad, happy, rich, or poor.

Terry has many interesting facets to his personality. He is a visionary leader, trusted partner, and a dear friend for all. His charisma and charm transcend all cultural and national barriers. Anyone who spends time with him will vouch for his in-depth understanding of human behavior.

Terry is passionate about natural health and is more than a motivational speaker. He is one of the leading proponents of natural health supplements I have ever come across in my career. Terry's thoughts on health, stress, life, diet, and natural remedies are on the cutting edge and a must for anyone committed to personal excellence.

The greatest gift that extraordinarily successful people have to give to others is their ability to motivate them to take action. And Terry's story is a testament to that. Terry's relentless passion to continually grow emotionally, socially, spiritually, and intellectually by staying positive and true to his ideals, makes him successful. And there is no doubt that it is his passion that has driven Terry to this elevated stature.

Great success is inseparable from the physical, intellectual, and spiritual energy that allows us to make the most of what we have. Terry uses many tools that can increase physical vibrancy.

I understand from Terry that things do not change; we have to change ourselves and focus on our goals, and our life becomes what we want it to be.

My association with Terry reminds me of Mark Twain's words, "There is no sadder sight than a young pessimist." People who believe in failure are certainly guaranteed a mediocre performance and existence. Terry does not believe in failure. In every set back, he sees an opportunity. People who achieve greatness don't dwell on what could go wrong but visualize what could go right. Terry's vision has touched so many uncounted lives and I am grateful to him for all he has done.

Introduction

WHY I WROTE THIS BOOK

Right now, we live in the United States of *Dis*-Ease. Diabetes, cancer, Alzheimer's, arthritis, and heart disease, to name only a few, are escalating. People are living longer, but with more illness and much less quality of life. We are selling more drugs, and spending more money on healthcare than at any point in the history of the human race, yet we as a nation are sicker than ever.

It is time to stop the madness. We are not going to cure our current ills with the next new pharmaceutical. Virtually all our health problems are linked to lifestyle choices and the disruption of how our bodies were meant to function. The answer is to change our lifestyle and use interventions to support our bodies, so they can once again function normally. This is where supplements and natural medicines shine and the reason I wanted to write this book. It's dedicated to guiding you on a journey to restoring good health, naturally.

I am not against modern medicine. If I get hit by a truck, I want to be taken to an emergency room trauma center with surgeons, nurses, and the most up-to-date hospital equipment. Mainstream medicine does trauma very well. However, when we look at the epidemic of modern diseases, chronic illnesses, and dysregulations, very few answers are forthcoming.

One of the biggest problems with modern medical practice is that it treats human beings like machines. But we're not machines. Our physical and mental health is intricately tied to our diets, level of exercise, relationships, spiritual life, environmental exposures, and many other factors too numerous to count.

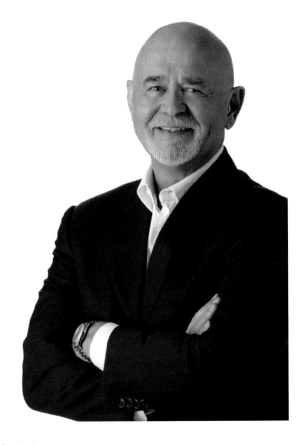

In the early 20th century, disease rates were very different from today. For example, cancer occurred in one person out of 25 a little over a hundred years ago. Today, cancer occurs in one out of two men and one out of three women.

Think about that for just a minute.

Researchers and scientists spend billions of dollars looking for cures for modern day diseases, like type 2 diabetes, that barely existed just 50 to 100 years ago. They look for quick synthetic, chemical fixes for problems that are rooted in our diet and lifestyle.

I know we can do better. There are natural, scientifically-validated ingredients that are much more successful than drugs, and without the dangers of severe side effects. I've put together this list of my top 50+ effective natural ingredients that can change lives and get us back on the right path to vibrant health.

My Own Health Story

Being addicted to an unhealthy lifestyle is easy. It's a set of habits into which any one of us can fall. I loved soda and candy, and had a very unhealthy diet. In fact, at one time in my teens and early 20s, at 5'7" tall, my weight ballooned to 250 pounds. It took being in the Marine Corps to keep me away from junk food. Also, my exercise routine (a daily obstacle course and 10-mile run) was "strongly encouraged," and I became healthier. I was fortunate to meet a captain in the Marine Corps who mentored me in

weight lifting and physical exercise, and introduced me to my first health food store in Oceanside, California.

The experience of healthy eating and regular physical exercise changed my life profoundly. I became a lifelong student of natural health, and eventually this became not only my passion, but my profession. I've worked over the past forty years to formulate and introduce hundreds of effective natural medicines to America. I've been an owner of health food stores and have created nutritional manufacturing companies. I was fortunate to introduce the concept of botanical standardization to the U.S. health food market after learning of its importance in Europe. I've been able to bring excellent products to America, including the introduction of glucosamine sulfate to our marketplace, IP-6 for cancer, and various complex formulations for specific health indications, including pain relief, preserving memory, and much more.

During my years in natural medicine, I've traveled the world, spoken with growers, researchers, and practitioners, and tried to absorb as much of their knowledge as possible. Along the way, my own health and the health of others with whom I've shared this information has improved as a result. It has been a wonderful experience.

The lifestyle that I adopted back in the Marine Corps eventually brought me to where I am today—healthy, at an appropriate weight, and with a better understanding about health and nutrition. It changed my whole life. Now I hope I can help you change your life.

HOW TO USE THIS BOOK

Each chapter discusses the powerful, proven health benefits of one of the top herbs I selected for this book. I briefly discuss the traditional use or origin of the ingredient, the major indications for its use as a natural medicine, a little bit about the scientific research, and how to choose the best form for optimal results. This last part is especially important. All herbal products are not created equal and can vary dramatically in important factors like safety, absorption, and key compounds. Buying the cheapest product from a dusty discount bin will not give you the results you need and will only leave you feeling disappointed. This book is not just a list of herbs, but a guidebook on how to use the very best, scientifically validated natural medicines to make a difference in your life.

Choosing Effective Supplements

So where do you start when choosing herbs? Do your homework. Start with clinical research. Of course, this book will answer some of your questions, but it's also important to use good scientific websites such as PubMed. If you intend to buy a product, call the manufacturer for additional questions. It's your health and you have a right to know what you are putting into your body.

Clinical Studies

The chapters in this book reference many scientific studies. My best advice to you is that if your interest is piqued by a certain scientific study, make sure you search for the exact plant the study was referencing. For example, there are some phenomenal studies being done on the ability of small molecular sized OPCs in French grape seed extract to suppress tumors and fight cancer. But inexpensive, high molecular tannins found in inexpensive grape seed extract is never going to have those same cancer-preventing abilities. You need to find the particular product or ingredients used in the studies to reap the same amazing benefits. So my first suggestion is to look for the exact clinically studied dietary supplement you read about.

Same Name, Different Benefits

It's also important to know that just because plants have the same name, it doesn't mean they'll provide the same therapeutic benefits. Yes, it's usually true that plants with the same name have the same composition of naturally-occurring phytonutrients. However, those phytonutrients are present in different concentrations based on where the plant is grown and how it's extracted. The environment where a plant is grown ultimately creates the plant, just like the environment we live in creates us. You and I are the same species; we're all human. But we vary as much as plants do based on the environments in which we live.

For example, echinacea grown in Bulgaria is different than echinacea grown in the United States, because of the varied environmental factors to which they've been exposed. These two types of echinacea weren't grown in the same type of soil with the same degree of moisture or the same exposure to sunshine. Therefore, they won't deliver equal benefits.

There's a scientific method to the culture of plants, and in some places—Europe, for example—they take the science of plant harvesting very seriously in the name of creating quality natural medicines. Plants have a higher concentration of nutrients at a specific time of the day, so some are harvested in the morning, some in the evening; it all depends on the plant. Many of my favorite products come from Europe because they focus on the best ways to cultivate plants to create formulas backed by science.

You Really Get What You Pay for in Most Cases

Another thing to keep in mind when choosing products is that price often dictates quality when it comes to dietary supplements. A health conscious supplement consumer won't make a purchase based simply on price. Let's look at echinacea again, for example. Say you read an amazing study on echinacea and head to your local health food store to make a purchase. When you get there, you're met with 25 different echinacea products on the shelves to sort through. The vast amount of products to choose from can be overwhelming: how do you make the right choice? Most people will purchase one of the less expensive options. Shopping by price alone is a poor way to choose dietary supplements. In order to keep prices low, cuts must be made to manufacturing standards and the quality of the raw materials. Most inexpensive products aren't going to work, and by trying one of these, you'll assume all echinacea don't' work for you. That is unfortunate, because the higher quality echinacea most likely will.

Create a Healthy Partnership

If you're still unsure where to start when searching for a specific extract, head straight to your local health food store. It's a much better source for supplements than generic "big box" stores, because health food stores have a mission in mind: to help people live better, naturally. Many of the products you're likely to find at discount stores were created with the idea of making money—not providing real ingredients you need at levels that matter.

Also, don't be afraid to contact the companies that make these supplements. Talk to someone there who can answer your questions about their ingredients and clinical research. The best supplement companies will be happy to form a relationship with their customers.

In the meantime, I hope you find this book informative and easy to read. You can read it from the first page to the last, or select chapters on herbal medicines in which you are particularly interested. However you choose to use this book, it is my sincerest hope that it provides you with the information you need to make a difference in your health, or the health of someone you love.

Amla/Indian Gooseberry: Boosts Protective HDL Cholesterol

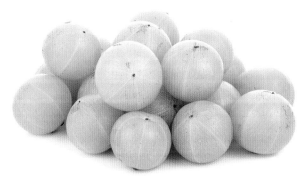

Amla, also known as Indian Gooseberry, has been used in Ayurvedic practice for over 2,000 years. Practitioners noted that it helped reduce inflammation, rebuild tissues throughout the body, make bones stronger, and strengthen vision.

· ·

Healthy Cholesterol Balance

Amla has more recently been the subject of intensive research for its ability to inhibit cancer growth in cervical cancer cells, melanoma cells, and human lung cells. One of the ways it can do this is simply through its intense antioxidant power. Amla can increase levels of the enzyme glutathione-S-transferase (GST), which detoxifies carcinogens from the body. It also boosts cancer-fighting NK (natural killer) cell activity and prevents DNA mutations caused by aluminum, lead, and chromium.

While amla can benefit the body in many ways, my favorite thing about it is its ability to get cholesterol levels in balance. I don't believe that cholesterol is the "enemy." In fact, cholesterol is crucial to our health. It's essential for healthy brain function, required for the maintenance of sex hormones, and necessary for the metabolism of fat-soluble vitamins in the body.

Having problematic imbalances in the types of cholesterol can be extremely dangerous and can contribute to oxidation and inflammation—the root of all disease in the body. Most serious cholesterol problems are due to not having enough HDL (high-density lipoprotein) or "good" cholesterol, which sets the stage for elevated LDL (low-density lipoproteins) or "bad" cholesterol. Thankfully, amla can help to get both of those numbers into their ideal range.

One clinical study showed that participants taking 500–1,000 mg of amla before bedtime increased HDL by 14 percent and significantly decreased LDL by 21 percent. Within three months, total cholesterol was reduced by 17 percent and triglyceride levels dropped by 24 percent. These numbers are extremely impressive because raising HDL levels by even one percent can reduce the risk of heart disease by two to three percent. The higher the HDL, the healthier the heart.

One form of Amla that is a whole fruit and seed extract is a raw material called Trilow.

DOSAGE RECOMMENDATIONS

I recommend starting with the clinically studied upper level of 1,000 mg daily. Choose an Amla fruit extract that is standardized to at least 35% polyphenol content.

THE CHOLESTEROL MYTH

There's a huge myth in our culture that cholesterol causes heart disease. This is simply not true, though many medical professionals still believe it. To defend this myth, many people have been sold a lot of misinformation and dangerous prescription drugs, creating a disaster for the nation's health.

When it comes to heart disease, the real problems are oxidation and inflammation. If we can safely and effectively stop these underlying causes of disease; we can get serious about eliminating preventable heart disease in this country. A good way to do that is by taking 1,000 mg of amla per day, which is proven to balance cholesterol levels and prevent oxidation.

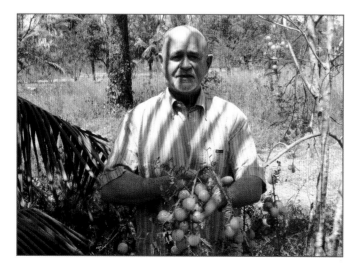

Terry in India, picking fresh Amla fruit, a time-honored Ayurvedic botanical.

Andrographis: The Crowning Jewel for Your Immune System

To some, andrographis (*Andrographis paniculata*) may not be well known, but this herb has been widely used in Ayurvedic medicine since ancient times in India, and Asia, and is currently used worldwide. Known as the "King of Bitters" because of its bitter taste, the herb is cultivated as an annual plant and grows up to three feet tall. While it has been recommended over the centuries for many purposes, I'd like to emphasize its application to stop colds, flu, and other infections.

A Royal Botanical

We have a great need for *effective* immune boosting interventions that don't create side effects. Also crucial—we need alternative, effective ways of protecting ourselves other than with antibiotics, which are quickly becoming obsolete and ineffective from decades of overuse and abuse.

Shortens Duration of Colds and Flu

Andrographis helps prevent the common cold, *and* reduces the intensity of symptoms, particularly sore throat and runny nose. Best of all, the research backs up these claims.

In a double-blind, placebo-controlled study, andrographis relieved the intensity of key symptoms in just *two* days. That included fatigue, sore throat, runny nose, and the sleeplessness that accompanies a cold. By the fourth day, there was a significant decrease in *all* symptoms, which included headache, earache, phlegm production, and the frequency and intensity of coughing spells.

Another clinical study of individuals with upper respiratory tract infection (URTI) showed similar results. In this

case, 223 patients either received 200 mg per day of andrographis or a placebo. At first, the results between the two seemed about the same. But by the third day, there was a dramatic difference in cough, headache, sore throat, and disturbed sleep. People in the placebo group noticed no improvement—in fact, some symptoms got worse—while those in the andrographis group saw a major difference in only five days.

For anyone who has ever dealt with colds, flu, or other upper respiratory infections that just won't go away, this is very good news. The fact that andrographis has no serious side effects makes it a much better choice than conventional options.

Aside from its cold and flu stopping power, scientific research shows that andrographis also protects the liver, regulates blood sugar levels, stops cancer cells from spreading, and acts as a strong anti-inflammatory. Because there are so many reasons to incorporate andrographis into your regimen, I consider it a "must have" herbal ingredient for everyone.

DOSAGE RECOMMENDATIONS

I would recommend 400 mg of andrographis leaf and stem extracts, providing a total of 80 mg of andrographolides per day.

Angelica Archangelica: Iceland's Bladder Botanical

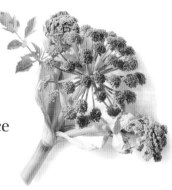

Icelandic Angelica, more properly known as *Angelica archangelica*, is found throughout the island nation. But even though it is commonplace, it is also exceptional and has been considered a valuable herb for over a thousand years. In fact, the Vikings once used it as currency, and Iceland's first book of law specifically banned theft of the plant.

• •

Historically, all the parts of the Angelica plant have been used—very often for its tonic value in restoring strength following illness. These days, modern research has been exploring the use of Angelica leaf extract to address a variety of common bladder problems.

Overactive Bladder, Common with Age

About 17 percent of women and 16 percent of men over the age of 18 have over-active bladder issues. As we age, overactive bladder becomes more common, affecting one in five adults over the age of 40.

For men, the causes of overactive bladder often overlap with symptoms of benign prostate hyperplasia (BPH). Also, pressure from the enlarging prostate on the bladder can reduce bladder capacity. Many men deal with nocturia—a need to go to the bathroom several times at night. And of course, the chances of being affected by nocturia increase with age for women, too.

Many others deal with daily stress incontinence, especially women, who worry that every sneeze or laugh will put too much pressure on their bladders and allow some degree of urine leakage.

But overall, urinary incontinence, whether due to chronic bladder irritation, bladder weakness, bacteria, or BPH, affects at least 25 million Americans. Most of the sufferers are women, but one-third of women *and* men 30 to 70 years old have experienced some symptoms of urinary incontinence.

A Better Bladder Means Better Sleep

And while bed-wetting is often associated with children, there are some adults who, because of their overactive or weak bladders, have *never* experienced a dry night.

Of course, one of the biggest problems with nocturia isn't just the fact of having to go to the bathroom; it's the disruption of sleep, and the low energy and grogginess the next day. After a while, the lack of sleep wears down immune resistance, reduces your ability to concentrate, leads to weight gain, and truly hurts your quality of life.

There are a few things that are measured when researchers test those dealing with nocturia, including nocturnal urinary output and nocturnal urinary capacity. What often happens as people age (and also in many cases of diabetes, BPH, and cardiovascular issues) is that bladder capacity decreases. This is because the bladder never seems to stop contracting, so there is less room in the bladder at any given time. Bladder tissue also gets weaker with age, making people more prone to accidental "leaks" before they can find a bathroom or while they sleep.

Icelandic Angelica Research

Improving bladder health is where Icelandic Angelica shines. This herb contains a number of important compounds, including one called isoquercitrin, along with a host of other flavonoids, polyphenols, and polysaccharides. These compounds are considered to be responsible for the plant's many beneficial effects. Some scientists believe that the intense arctic summer—with 24 hours of daylight—spurs the growth and concentration of nutrients in this plant.

In an eight-week, randomized, double-blind, placebo-controlled study, men over the age of 45 suffering from nocturia received Angelica leaf extract or placebo. During this study, three main parameters were measured: the increase in bladder volume, reduction in getting up at night to urinate, and the increase in the duration of the first sleep period before first awakened by urinary pressure. The results were excellent.

- In the subgroup with low bladder capacity, those taking Angelica saw an increase of over 300 percent in bladder capacity.

- In the subgroup with more than three urinary voids during the night, Angelica reduced voids by as much as 50 percent.

- And, in the subgroup of men age 70 or older, Angelica increased the first uninterrupted sleep period almost three fold vs. the placebo group. This is impressive, because the prevalence of nocturia for men age 70 and older can range from 50 percent to 80 percent or more. No wonder so many older individuals only get a few hours of sleep each night.

This study showed that the direct action of Angelica was not on the prostate, but rather on the bladder. This means its benefits apply to both men and women, since it is not hormonal in its activity. Plus, it was very well tolerated and showed no serious adverse effects, no increased blood pressure or heart rate, or reduced libido—a definite difference from many prescription drugs.

So why does it work? Icelandic Angelica quiets the overstimulated nerves that create a sense of urgency in an overactive bladder. It helps reduce bladder inflammation and irritation, and it improves the ability of the bladder to hold a larger amount of urine comfortably. During the day, that means fewer trips to the bathroom and less urgency. At night, it means the same thing, plus better, undisturbed, and restful sleep.

While there are prescription drugs that address incontinence, many of them carry serious risks and side effects.

Risky Drugs Are Not the Answer

The class of drugs (anticholinergics known by brand names including Ditropan, Vesicare, and Detrol) used to treat overactive bladder have been found to cause cognitive impairment after only two months of use. They deplete the body of much-needed choline. Worse yet, if a person is using a drug for overactive bladder or incontinence, and then also takes an over the counter drug like Benadryl (diphenhydramine, also an anticholinergic) for allergies, or Advil PM, Tylenol PM, etc. for sleep, the potential for dementia is magnified.

This is not the case with Icelandic Angelica. It does not reduce choline or have any significant risks. That means you reap the benefits.

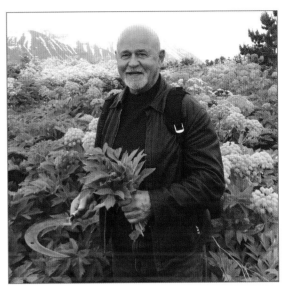

Terry picking Angelica in Iceland.

If you deal with an overactive bladder, a sense of urgency, or frequent trips to the bathroom at night, *Angelica archangelica* extract is an excellent choice. Use in the morning and again at night for the first few days, and then drop down to once per day when you start to notice a difference. Between the peace of mind, better sleep, and overall well-being you'll experience, Angelica can make a dramatic improvement to your life.

DOSAGE RECOMMENDATIONS

Starting out with just 200 mg per day for the first few days of use, and then tapering back to 100 mg per day can make a life-changing difference.

Aronia (Chokeberry): A Little-Known Superstar

Most people know the importance of seasonal berries as part of a healthy diet. However, when it comes to nutrition, most berries must take a back seat to aronia—the mighty chokeberry! This extensively researched, highly nutritious berry originates from a shrub native to North America. While it remains relatively unknown as an edible berry here in the U.S.A., it's an everyday staple in Eastern European countries like Poland and Russia.

Not only is aronia a hearty and attractive shrub, with white flowers in the spring that turn into berries in summer, it also provides a powerhouse of nutrients. The shrub grows from six to nine feet tall and produces a high abundance of berries—about 20 to 40 pounds per bush. Chokeberries are easy to pick, freeze well, and are an excellent addition to oatmeal, yogurt, jams, and jellies, or as the basis for juice or wine.

Not the Nicest Name

Chokeberry, or black chokeberry as it is called in different parts of the world, is not a very appetizing name for an edible berry. The name comes from its tart flavor, due to the tannins in the berries. The tannins produce an astringency in the mouth—a dry sensation similar to tasting a very dry wine. Unlike the sweetness found in blueberries and strawberries, the chokeberry is unpalatable to some people. Ironically, children, including my grandchildren, eat them by the handfuls with no problem. Adults usually end up with a "puckered" look on their face when they sample their first berry. They lean toward using them in a smoothie or sprinkled on a salad.

A Berry to Compare

Despite an unappetizing name, the big news about aronia is its nutritional value. A member of the family *Rosaceae*, aronia has an exceptionally high ORAC rating. ORAC units measure the antioxidant capacity of foods. The higher the ORAC score, the better. For comparison, a blueberry has an ORAC value of 4,669. A strawberry—4,302. Aronia, the chokeberry? 16,062! With high amounts of phenolic flavonoid phytochemicals called anthocyanins—antioxidants that have proven health benefits through scavenging dangerous free radicals from the body—the chokeberry is a great addition to anyone's daily diet.

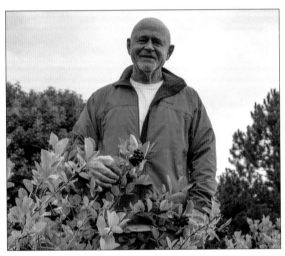

Terry in his backyard in Wisconsin, picking Aronia berries.

Just in Case

Aronia berries do contain oxalic acid, which naturally occurs in some fruits and vegetables. For a very small group of people, probably only one percent of the population, oxalic acid can crystallize as oxalate stones in the urinary tract. If you are the one percent, you may want to avoid chokeberries.

Aronia Close to Home

I usually travel the world to find botanicals, but when it comes to chokeberries, I merely need to step out into my yard. It all began when I received ten chokeberry bushes for my birthday a few years ago. I liked them so much; I added 60 more bushes. Even though over 80 pounds of chokeberries were gathered at my last picking, I've decided to add additional Aronia shrubs and plan for even more in the future. With the great harvest coming, there will be an Aronia version of wine in my future. Meanwhile, enjoy this recipe for adding Aronia to your next smoothie.

MY FAVORITE CHOKEBERRY PROTEIN DRINK

8 oz. organic milk or favorite beverage

$1/2$ cup Aronia berries

1 scoop of your favorite protein powder

$1/2$ banana

1 Tbsp almond butter

Ashwagandha:
A Strength and Stamina Marvel

Ashwagandha belongs to an elite group of botanicals called adaptogens. Adaptogens are one of my favorite groups of plants, because they have the unique ability to restore balance in the body.

With an extensive history of usage dating back thousands of years, ashwagandha has been a staple in the traditional medicinal system of India called Ayurveda. Historically, ashwagandha has been used to combat fatigue and improve stamina. Present-day research has validated these benefits, and also uncovered some of the biological mechanisms behind its power.

Stress and Health

Many people are under chronic stress, and whether it's work, family, financial, or environmental, it can have a negative impact on our health. One way in which stress can cause health problems is by the excessive release of the adrenal hormone cortisol. High levels of cortisol are associated with sleeplessness, nervousness, high blood sugar levels, and abdominal weight gain. In a 2016 study, people under chronic stress were given a standardized ashwagandha extract (KSM-66) or placebo, and then they evaluated negative parameters associated with stress, like overeating and food cravings. At the end of eight weeks, the ashwagandha group had significant reductions in weight, body mass index (BMI), cortisol levels, and food cravings. Additionally, a 2012 human study using the same ashwagandha extract also noted significant reductions in stress and cortisol levels.

Building Muscle

Even building muscle is physiologically stressful. It involves tearing muscle fibers, followed by a complex process of repair and growth. A study done on resistance training and recovery found that KSM-66 Ashwagandha significantly increased muscle strength while decreasing the biological markers of muscle injury. This means greater results from your workout, and less time spent repairing damage, so that more resources can be shifted to reaching your exercise goals.

The Fountain of Youth?

Another exciting area of ashwagandha research is longevity. While the fountain of youth is yet to be discovered, ashwagandha may be a key factor in slowing down the process of aging. In a scientific study, KSM-66 Ashwagandha was tested on human cells and found to increase the activity of an enzyme that protects the tail ends of our genes, called telomeres. By protecting the telomeres, our chromosomes can replicate more times. More replications is strongly associated with a longer lifespan.

Surviving Cancer

Ashwagandha also has numerous anti-cancer properties; it has been scientifically studied for its beneficial effects on ovarian, breast, prostate, head, neck, lymph, and liver cancer cells. Ashwagandha is cytotoxic, meaning it kills cancer cells, without having adverse effects on normal cells. It also helps to prevent angiogenesis—or the formation of new blood vessels that feed the tumor, and prevents tumors from metastasizing (spreading cancer to other parts of the body).

Ashwagandha improves the activation of genes that suppress tumors and helps to regulate a process called apoptosis, which is programmed cell death. Cancer cells do not respond normally to apoptosis, so they continue to live, grow, and replicate. When ashwagandha is introduced to these cells, they once again have a definitive lifespan, and behave more like normal cells.

DOSAGE RECOMMENDATIONS

The clinical trials on ashwagandha used a wide range of dosages, anywhere from 500 mg to 5 grams per day. For general maintenance and prevention purposes, I think 600 mg per day is sufficient. For more serious health conditions, it may be necessary to increase the dose. While the efficacy of ashwagandha extracts can vary greatly, I think it's important to choose an extract that is standardized to at least five percent withanolides, key compounds that are responsible for many of ashwagandha's benefits. KSM-66 is a clinically studied form of this herb that meets these specifications.

Astaxanthin: Pink Perfection

Astaxanthin may not be the most commonly known compound, but it *is* one of nature's most valuable.

It is a uniquely-structured carotenoid, in the same family as beta-carotene and lutein. Astaxanthin is found in many sources, including yeast, salmon, trout, krill, and shrimp, although one of the richest dietary sources of astaxanthin is from *Haematococcus pluvialis,* a freshwater form of green microalgae. Astaxanthin helps the microalgae by enhancing the activity of chlorophyll to create food and energy from sunlight. Astaxanthin helps protect the microalgae from the damaging effects of free radicals, which is exactly what it does for us, too.

Surprisingly, astaxanthin renders a pinkish hue to the creatures that consume foods rich in this antioxidant. That is why salmon and shrimp have pink colorations. It is also why flamingos are so brilliantly colored!

• •

Nature's Perfect Compound

Astaxanthin is strong. It can help keep your heart and blood vessels healthy, provide critical DNA support, improve athletic performance and recovery by reducing oxidative stress and lactic acid, protect the delicate retinal structures of the eyes, and prevent damage throughout the body.

Loving Your Heart

Clinical and scientific research backs up the benefits of astaxanthin. For instance, a Japanese study showed that supplementation with astaxanthin for 12 weeks boosted HDL cholesterol (commonly called "good cholesterol") levels, reduced triglycerides, and increased adiponectin—a protein involved with the breakdown of fatty acids and the ability of the body to deal with blood sugar.

Boosts Endurance

Astaxanthin also improves our physical endurance, exercise recovery, and fat burning. It does this by helping the body use existing fat stores, rather than glucose, as an energy source during exercise, so you get more benefit from the exercise itself. Plus, research shows that this carotenoid reduces lactic acid in muscle tissue, so you'll experience less soreness, with the additional benefit of antioxidant and anti-inflammatory protection for your muscles.

Stops Eye Strain and Preserves Vision

For anyone who spends time on a computer —and that's many of us—astaxanthin is a perfect choice for keeping your eyes healthy. In a clinical study, it reduced eye strain by 54 percent in just one month. Astaxanthin also protects the delicate structure of the eyes and may help strengthen blood vessels in the retina. It has also been combined with other antioxidants and compounds for dry eye treatment, so I can't recommend it enough for a person

experiencing eye fatigue and soreness, or simply as a preventative measure to preserve focus and vision.

Brain Friendly and More

Astaxanthin from *Haematococcus pluvialis* has been shown to improve cognitive performance for individuals aged 45 to 64 who had complained of mild memory loss. By the end of the 12-week, placebo-controlled study, a dose of six mg per day helped people improve scores on a variety of memory-related tests. Not surprisingly, doubling the dose showed even greater results.

Other research is showing that astaxanthin may help fight liver damage and boost key immune system markers, making it a must-have ingredient during cold and flu season.

Uniquely Structured Compound

One of the reasons that astaxanthin is so powerful is due to the structure of the compound. It can actually work both inside and outside of a cell wall—keeping oxidative damage at bay and preventing it from entering a cell—while helping stop damage to the inside of a cell membrane at the same time. In fact, one study found that it was twice as effective as beta-carotene. Astaxanthin is also both fat- and water-soluble, which essentially doubles its absorption and capabilities.

Astaxanthin is probably the healthiest compound most people have never heard of. But now that you have, I urge you to incorporate it into your regimen every day—it can work wonders for your health!

DOSAGE RECOMMENDATIONS

The good news is that you don't need massive doses of astaxanthin to optimize your health. I believe 4–12 mg per day is a beneficial dose range.

Black Cohosh: Menopause and More

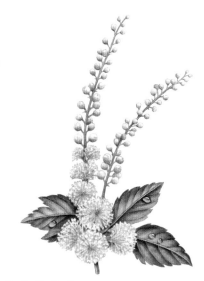

Every day, millions of women arrive at a time in their life when they wonder what they should do about the irritations caused by perimenopause and menopause. From hot flashes to mood swings, from night sweats to sleeplessness, menopause can rob a woman of what should be a time of wisdom and enjoyment. Fortunately, there is a proven, clinically studied answer to deal with that bothersome question, "Why is it so hot in here?"

• • • • • • • • • • • • • • • • • •

A Natural Choice

After the much publicized, potential long-term risks associated with standard hormone replacement therapy (HRT), including the danger of serious consequences like an increased possibility of breast cancer and stroke, many women are interested in a natural choice for menopausal symptom relief. One of the best natural options available is black cohosh, an herb with a long history of medicinal use. Used as a home remedy in 19th-century America and even before that by Native Americans, black cohosh is native to North America and is a member of the buttercup family (**Actaea racemose**) For more than five decades, black cohosh has been used throughout Europe for women's discomfort including menopausal symptoms.

Clinically Proven Benefits

Black cohosh's effectiveness has been proven in clinical research. In a controlled study of 629 women with menopausal complaints, 76 to 93 percent of those taking a standardized extract of black cohosh twice a day had an overall improvement in hot flashes, headache, irritability, heart palpitations, mild depression, and sleep disturbances. Another study of 120 women with menopausal symptoms reported that black cohosh was more effective in relieving hot flashes and night sweats than the antidepressant fluoxetine (Prozac). These are just a few of the many studies done on black cohosh.

Choose Black Cohosh Carefully

Not all black cohosh is created equal. In fact, some black cohosh isn't even black cohosh, as demonstrated by the recent scandal showing some black cohosh raw material was not even the correct species. Some companies are using Asian Cimicifuga in the preparation instead of black cohosh, so make sure you work with companies you trust.

Choosing an effective black cohosh comes down to paying attention to important details regarding the type of black cohosh you choose. The concentration, standardization, and dosage levels matter. Black cohosh may be the answer you need to journey through menopause comfortably and without prescription drugs.

DOSAGE RECOMMENDATIONS

European clinical studies have shown that an effective dose is 13 mg a day of the extract. One last thing to remember: it's important to take black cohosh for a minimum of three months before evaluating the results.

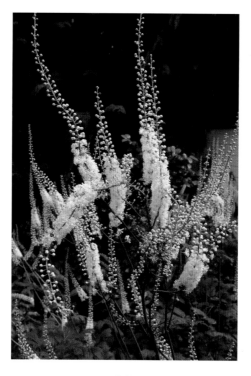

Boswellia/Frankincense: A Gift Suited for a King

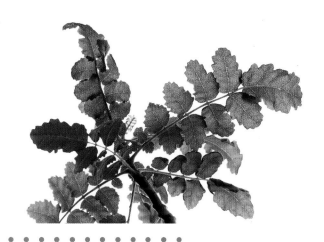

Boswellia is one of nature's most powerful anti-inflammatory medicines. In fact, research shows that it can effectively treat a wide variety of conditions, including asthma, allergies, arthritis, irritable bowel syndrome, Crohn's disease, celiac disease, and even cancer.

Native to India, the boswellia tree secretes a resin commonly known as frankincense. While the use of this resin dates back thousands of years, it is only in recent decades that it has been clinically studied for its amazing health benefits. Boswellia is believed to combat pain, relieve respiratory distress, protect the cardiovascular system, stop digestive diseases, and prevent tumors. How does the resin from one tree do so much? It all comes down to its ability to inhibit an enzyme called 5-lipoxygenase (5-LOX) that activates certain hard-to-treat inflammation in the body.

Look for 10% Naturally Occurring AKBA

Prescription medications usually only act on one enzymatic pathway, but natural compounds like boswellia contain phytonutrients that exert a multitude of therapeutic effects throughout the body. And although other herbal compounds relieve inflammation, none of them work on the 5-LOX pathway as well as boswellia. Boswellia contains compounds called boswellic acids that work directly to extinguish 5-LOX inflammation. The most active of these boswellic acids is known as Acetyl-11-keto-ß boswellic acids. That is certainly a mouthful! So it is much easier to refer to its nickname, AKBA. The most effective boswellia extracts contain at least 10% of naturally occurring AKBA. Also, boswellia contains beta boswellic acid or BBA. This boswellic acid actually causes inflammation, so the best boswellia products are purified to greatly reduce this compound.

Breathe Easy

For those suffering from respiratory ailments, boswellia can offer relief by opening airways, reducing bronchial and sinus swelling, and lessening allergy symptoms. This was shown in a double-blind, placebo-controlled clinical trial involving 40 patients with bronchial asthma. Each patient took either 300 mg of boswellia three times a day or a placebo for six weeks. By the end of the study, 70 percent of those taking the boswellia showed marked improvement compared to just 27 percent in the placebo group.

Many of the same triggers that cause asthma also cause allergies and chronic sinusitis. Fortunately, scientific studies report that boswellia can inhibit the action of mast cells, which are the culprits that release excessive amounts of histamine. Histamine causes congestion, irritation, watery eyes, sneezing and lots of mucus production.

Boswellia may also benefit those struggling with chronic obstructive pulmonary disease (COPD) or emphysema. Preliminary research suggests that the herb specifically inhibits a white blood cell that triggers respiratory symptoms in those with emphysema or chronic bronchitis. This may reduce the sensation of not being able to take a full breath or the feeling of "drowning" experienced by those with COPD. Also, by effectively relieving inflammation in the lungs, better air exchange occurs.

Improve Inflammatory Bowel

Boswellia has also been found to be extremely effective for patients dealing with IBS, Crohn's Disease, and ulcerative colitis. An Italian study examined boswellia serrate for its anti-inflammatory and anti-oxidant properties in patients with various inflammatory bowel diseases. When used proactively, boswellia helped to protect intestinal epithelial cells from inflammatory damage.

In another study in Germany, individuals with Crohn's disease were treated with boswellia or a drug called mesalazine, which is commonly used to treat patients with severe intestinal disorders. Boswellia performed equally as well as mesalazine, but caused none of the dangerous side effects that are often associated with use of prescription drugs.

Relieve Joint Pain

Perhaps boswellia is best known for its ability to treat pain, especially when it's combined with curcumin. Together, these two natural compounds reduce the activity of all the inflammatory pathways in the body, which in turn greatly reduces pain. They are so effective in combination, they were judged to be superior to the prescription drug celecoxib in a clinical trial of osteoarthritis. Sixty-four percent of those taking the herbal ingredients verses 29 percent in the drug group reported such significant pain relief that they were moved from having "moderate to severe arthritis" to "mild to moderate" arthritis.

DOSAGE RECOMMENDATIONS

A standard dosing recommendation for boswellia is 500–1,000 mg daily. If you are treating a specific inflammatory condition, a higher dose may be needed. Make sure the boswellia supplement you choose is standardized so you're getting at least 10% AKBA.

UNDERSTANDING INFLAMMATION

The body's inflammatory response keeps you healthy and safe from a wide range of illnesses and injuries. Acute inflammation is a short-term healing process that usually only lasts 24 to 48 hours. The goal of inflammation is to increase blood flow to the injured area, which helps immune cells enter the damaged tissue and initiate the healing process. This can be a tricky situation, though, because those same cells, systems, and enzymes needed to alleviate pain and inflammation can contribute to chronic internal inflammation, with dangerous ramifications.

Trouble begins when acute inflammation doesn't subside. When inflammation becomes chronic, it's like a slow, silent disturbance that never shuts off. Ongoing research suggests that chronic low-level inflammation throughout the body is involved in arthritis, Alzheimer's disease, cancer, cardiovascular disease, depression, diabetes, and other serious illnesses. Fortunately, natural anti-inflammatories like standardized boswellia can help quench the fires of chronic inflammation when taken on a daily basis.

Butcher's Broom:
For Better Legs

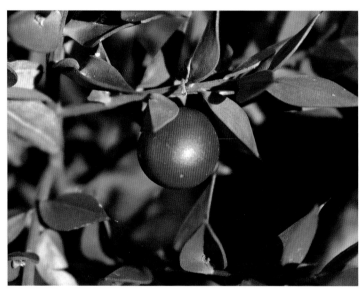

If you've noticed varicose veins and a tired, heavy feeling and swelling in your legs, you may have chronic venous insufficiency, also known as CVI. This happens because the veins in your legs have lost some of their natural ability to pump blood back up toward the heart. The valves that used to help push blood upward, back to the heart, have either become weakened or in some cases, have failed altogether. And that swelling you may have noticed is actually blood and other fluids pooling in the veins.

• •

A Vein-Saving Herb

Butcher's broom (*Ruscus aculeatus*) is native to Europe and North Africa. The root of the plant is the source of many beneficial compounds, ruscogenin being one of the most important.

Although well known in folk medicine, butcher's broom is also recognized as an effective herb by the German Commission E monographs, a body of botanical knowledge that is considered one of the premier authorities on natural medicine.

Proven Power

Clinical research investigating butcher's broom has found impressive results. One placebo-controlled trial wanted to confirm how effective butcher's broom extract truly was for chronic venous insufficiency. In fact, the researchers very deliberately wanted to use the same standards for butcher's broom as was used in conventional drugs to treat the same condition. The study focused on important measurements: leg volume changes, circumference of the lower leg and ankle, plus subjective symptoms including quality of life, overall effectiveness, and tolerability.

In only eight weeks, significant improvements were seen in leg volume and ankle and leg circumferences. By 12 weeks, leg volume was reduced even further, and the heaviness and tension in the legs had noticeably improved, too. Butcher's broom extract was clearly helping the veins in the legs pump blood back up toward the heart, and because of this, the subjective symptoms—the feelings about quality of life make CVI so tough to live with—became better as well. Best of all, butcher's broom was well-tolerated, without serious adverse effects.

Whether tested alone or in combination with other ingredients, butcher's broom repairs our delicate circulatory machinery, and acts as a strong anti-inflammatory. Butcher's broom may also help individuals suffering from chronic orthostatic hypotension (OH), a condition of low blood pressure that makes people feel dizzy when standing, which affects people with diabetes, Parkinson's and chronic fatigue syndrome. It is a very effective natural medicine.

If you work on your feet or notice bruising, fatigue, and heaviness in your legs, butcher's broom is a must for your daily regimen.

DOSAGE RECOMMENDATIONS

Dosage levels of butcher's broom have varied greatly, and you'll see capsules with up to 500 mg of the extract. However, the important thing to look for is a standardization of at least 10 percent ruscogenin content.

Cat's Claw:
An Amazonian Wonder

Cat's claw is one of the gifts from the Amazon rain forest that has been used for generations. From relieving joint pain to enhancing the body's defense in multiple areas, cat's claw is the answer. With curved, claw-like thorns all along its stem, cat's claw is a climbing vine that grows mostly in Central and South America. Originally discovered and used by the Inca civilization, the stories of what cat's claw accomplished caused scientists to study this wonder of the jungle.

• •

A Powerful Medicine

A rich source of phytochemicals with 30-plus constituents, cat's claw (*Uncaria tomentosa*) includes at least 17 alkaloids and other phytonutrients that contribute to its powerful health benefits. However, cat's claw comes in two variants. One form provides medicinal compounds called pentacyclic oxindole alkaloids (POAs), while the other provides ineffective tetracyclic oxindole alkaloids (TOAs). If the herb is not standardized to be only the POA form, you may not receive any benefits at all!

Cat's Claw Uses

Cat's claw is that rarest of herbs—it is a true immune system modulator. That means if your immune system is misbehaving, as in an autoimmune disease, it will help it to slow down and behave more normally. If your immune system is weakened, it will help the body fortify its immune activity by boosting t-cell (a kind of white blood cell) production and activity.

The POA form of cat's claw has been clinically studied for rheumatoid arthritis, the most common autoimmune disease in America. One study found that when people taking sulfasalazine or hydroxychloroquine—two drugs commonly used to treat RA—added in cat's claw, they had fewer painful, swollen joints than those who took a placebo. Research also suggests a decrease in inflammation for those with osteoarthritis.

Because of its ability to improve t-cell levels, the POA form of cat's claw has also been used by people who are HIV positive or who have AIDS. It is important to note, however, that early research indicates that cat's claw may increase the levels of HIV drugs called antiretrovirals in the body. While this may be useful in some situations, it is important to work with your healthcare practitioner to monitor the most optimal ways to combine supplements with mainstream medical interventions.

Cat's claw is also useful for people who are concerned about cancer due to its specific antioxidant and antitumor activity. Cat's claw inhibits the activation of nuclear factor-kappa beta, an inflammatory "switch" associated with cancer, and other deadly diseases linked to chronic low-level inflammation and immune system dysfunction. AIDS, Alzheimer's, Lyme Disease, Crohn's Disease, asthma, ulcers… the list keeps growing for the conditions that can benefit from cat's claw.

Cat's Claw Cautions and Future

Make sure your cat's claw is standardized to contain 1.3 percent pentacyclic oxindole alkaloids (POAs) and free of tetracyclic oxindole alkaloids (TOAs.) You want to use a product with the plant source of *uncaria tomentosa* and not *uncaria guianensis*. These species are sometimes confused.

Research continues to uncover more uses for cat's claw. With its benefits exceeding most known immune enhancing or modulating herbs—including reishi, echinacea, eleuthero (formerly known as Siberian ginseng), and astragalus—we will keep discovering more about this amazing treasure from the Amazon rainforest.

DOSAGE RECOMMENDATIONS

Take a 20 mg capsule three times daily for the first ten days, and one capsule daily after that.

Chasteberry:
A Woman's Good Friend

With an estimated 85 percent of menstruating women having at least one PMS symptom as part of their monthly cycle, it's no wonder that ladies are looking for an answer for the food cravings, bloating, trouble sleeping, breast pain, cramps, mood swings, and depression that can be a part of PMS. Research points to clinically studied chasteberry as a natural solution.

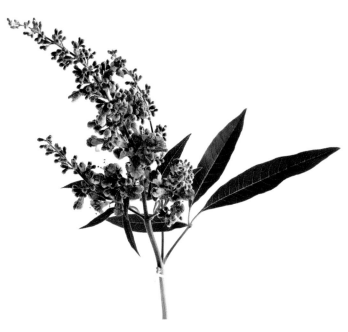

Women Through the Ages

Dating back to ancient Greek times, women have relied on chasteberry (*Vitex agnus castus*) to ease the symptoms of premenstrual syndrome and menopause. This herb is also known as vitex, chaste tree berry, and monk's pepper. Today we know that chasteberry contains a wealth of phytochemicals including flavonoids, essential oils, diterpenes, and glycosides.

Chasteberry works by balancing hormones released by the pituitary gland. Scientific studies show that chasteberry may affect dopamine (a neurotransmitter involved in regulating emotional responses and suppressing prolactin release). Lowering prolactin levels can result in an increase in progesterone. Most women with PMS have decreased progesterone production two weeks before menstruation, and chasteberry is very useful in boosting progesterone levels into a healthier range.

Proof for PMS

Results from clinical studies on chasteberry have been impressive, showing it to be effective for most PMS complaints. In one randomized, placebo-controlled study, 170 women were divided into treatment and placebo groups, with the treatment group given 20 mg of standardized chasteberry extract over three consecutive menstrual cycles. Compared to the placebo group, those taking the chasteberry experienced significant relief, especially for irritability, mood swings, anger, headache, and breast fullness. Overall, the authors noted that over half of the women in the chasteberry group had a 50 percent or greater improvement in their PMS symptoms.

Dosage Matters

When it comes to chasteberry, more is not better. In one 2012 study, participants who were given 30 mg of chasteberry extract did not show greater improvement in symptoms than those in the 20 mg group. A 2014 study examined over 20 different chasteberry products and found wide variation in the key components of chasteberry, such as casticin. Some were too low to be clinically effective, and some were too high, which can point to adulteration with other chasteberry species.

If you are suffering from the difficult physical and emotional problems of PMS, try a safe alternative for relief: chasteberry. But be sure to give it at least three months to work. Some women will feel results earlier, but clinical trials show that ongoing use of chasteberry extract for several weeks is necessary for a therapeutic effect.

DOSAGE RECOMMENDATIONS

It's best to opt for 20 mg a day of a 6:1 extract—6:1 means that it takes 120 mg of the dried herb to make 20 mg of extract.

Cherry Fruit:
For Gout and More

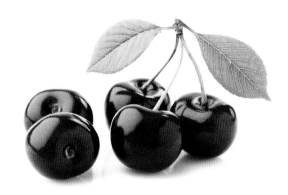

Cherries are a sweet, flavorful fruit, but have also been shown by researchers to be an antioxidant powerhouse with the ability to prevent or treat injuries and disease.

Cherry's Secret

There are actually two distinct types of cherries—sweet and tart. While all cherries provide some health benefits, studies suggest that it's the less palatable tart cherry that is packed with more plant pigments called anthocyanins. The anthocyanins are what provide the cherry's powerful antioxidant and anti-inflammatory properties. Anythocyanins reduce oxidative stress and damage to DNA (a risk factor for cancer). They also reduce levels of uric acid, a compound in the blood that can cause a gout attack. Tart cherry is beneficial for a wide variety of diseases and conditions. They even reduce the risk of type 2 diabetes.

Good for Gout

While there is no cure for gout, a type of arthritis that results in a painful uric acid build-up in the blood and crystallization in the joints, multiple studies show that tart cherry extract can be an answer for the severe pain and inflammation of this troubling disease. One study published in 2010 looked at the use of cherry juice in marathon runners. In this study, participants were given tart cherry juice or placebo juice daily for seven days before a marathon and on race day. The researchers measured muscle damage, inflammatory markers (including uric acid levels), and oxidative stress before and after the race. Those who took the cherry juice experienced faster strength recovery and reduced inflammatory markers compared to those in the placebo group.

Another study on tart cherries for gout published in *Arthritis* in 2012 showed that tart cherry juice concentrate was able to inhibit inflammatory markers in cells, demonstrating tart cherry's potent anti-inflammatory effects. A 2014 clinical study examined the effects of tart cherry juice on blood levels of uric acid and inflammatory markers in healthy volunteers. The researchers found that those who drank cherry juice for two days had significantly reduced levels of uric acid and the inflammatory marker C-reactive protein in their blood.

Juice or Supplement?

So, why not just drink tart cherry juice? Because you probably wouldn't like it!

Tart cherries are very sour and need quite a bit of sugar to make the juice palatable. With a supplement, you get the tart cherry benefits without the sugar load. In one cherry juice concentrate, just two tablespoons contained 80 calories from sugar.

Since there are multiple extraction methods used in the preparation of tart cherry supplements, look for one that uses freeze-drying technology, and has no added sugar. Extraction methods other than freeze-drying can result in a 35 to 75 percent depletion of the valuable nutrients you seek.

DOSAGE RECOMMENDATIONS

Choose a quality freeze-dried cherry supplement in the convenient capsule form with 750 mg of tart cherry fruit powder per capsule. Take one or two capsules twice a day for best results.

GETTING YOUR ZZZ'S AND TART CHERRY

Try tart cherry for help with sleeping. In a 2012 study, those taking a tart cherry concentrate showed an increase in melatonin—a molecule found in regulating the sleep-wake cycle and a phytochemical found in tart cherries. Compared to the placebo group, those taking the tart cherry concentrate had significant increases in total sleep time, time in bed, and more efficient sleep. This doesn't mean you can't take tart cherry in the daytime—it won't make you sleepy. But by building your body's store of melatonin, your nights will be more restful and restorative.

Comfrey:
Botanical Comfort and Healing

If we could visit apothecaries hundreds, or even thousands of years ago, no doubt we would have found comfrey on hand for numerous health conditions. The whole plant—root, leaves, and flowers—has been used medicinally in many cultures throughout history. Even 2000 years ago, its effects on broken bones were recorded.

The Latin name for comfrey, *Symphytum officinale*, has a translation that means to heal or join together, and historic names for comfrey included boneknit, boneset, and bruisewort. In most recent studies, comfrey is used topically in an easily absorbed cream. Not only can this botanical shorten the duration of healing for fractures, sprains, strains, but it can also help with superficial wound injuries like burns and skin abrasions.

Comfrey Research

Recent comfrey research has reaffirmed what our ancestors have known for millennia. However, scientists also discovered that traditionally-used comfrey contains harmful compounds called pyrrolizidine alkaloids (PA), which can damage the liver.

In fact, oral comfrey products and teas are no longer sold in the United States, although its use in topical creams and ointments has continued to be allowed. Fortunately, a natural medicine company in Germany has developed a cultivar of comfrey that delivers all the benefits but does NOT contain these harmful PA compounds. It is the first, and so far, only company to do so. Because this specific comfrey is PA-free, you can apply it to broken skin without worry. This unique comfrey has been researched for its effects on ankle and knee sprains, tendon injuries, chronic back and neck pain, muscle damage and soreness, pressure ulcers, and wound healing in adults and children.

Safe for Children

When children play a little too rough, or fall off their bike; there aren't a lot of safe and effective options to relieve their pain and speed their healing. But comfrey cream can do both—which is why I think it is such a great natural medicine. A clinical study with over 190 children, ages 4–12 years old, used a topical comfrey cream to treat strains and sprains. The comfrey cream relieved pain, swelling, and bruising—without any side effects. In 2012, a clinical study with over 100 children ages 3–12 years old, tested comfrey's effects on fresh abrasions (a high-dose comfrey preparation vs. low-dose comfrey preparation). The high-dose group healed 50 percent faster than children in the low-dose treatment group. But here again, neither group experienced any side effects. Comfrey's unique anti-inflammatory properties make it perfect for relieving bug bites, stings, rashes, burns, and acne, too.

Comfrey shows results for adults as well. If you've ever felt sidelined from your exercise regimen because of soreness and pain, comfrey can help you stay on track. In a clinical study on exercise-induced muscle soreness, comfrey was shown to reduce pain in just 15 minutes. It is the ideal natural medicine to keep in your gym or yoga bag. Another study examined comfrey cream's effects on sports-related injuries to the knee, including sprains and bruising. Of the 40 patients in the comfrey group, 85 percent rated its effects as good or very good. And 100 percent found no side effects or problems with tolerability. That's pretty rare in a topical.

Back Pain and More

Back pain common? Chances are, you've dealt with it due to exercise, household chores, or as part of your job. You may be tempted to self-medicate with over-the-counter pain relievers. Unfortunately, these solutions can cause gastrointestinal bleeding and ulcers, liver and kidney issues, and even dull your emotions. Comfrey cream is a better alternative. In a study involving 215 people with upper and lower back pain, a PA-free comfrey cream significantly reduced pain in motion, at rest, or from hands-on examination by a physician. And again, these powerful results came without the risk of harmful side effects.

How to Use Comfrey

Comfrey is a botanical that has truly withstood the test of time. While traditional usage includes comfrey compresses, teas, tinctures, and salves, the comfrey preparation I prefer is a cream made from the freshly pressed aerial parts of the German comfrey plant. This specific type of comfrey can be used on open wounds because it is PA free, and is safe for the whole family—even pregnant women and nursing mothers! The clinical studies on this PA-free comfrey cream used anywhere from one to five applications per day.

DOSAGE RECOMMENDATIONS

The clinical studies on PA-free comfrey cream used anywhere from one to five applications per day. It is very safe, and you should use the amount to cover the area you wish to treat.

SAFETY MATTERS

Certain plant species contain compounds called *pyrrolizidine alkaloids* (PA), as part of their natural defenses. These compounds help protect the plant. Since they are unable to move, plants must synthesize protective chemicals to defend themselves from predators and pathogens. While comfrey is not the only plant that produces PA, its popularity in herbal medicine has greatly expanded its use throughout the world. In humans, excessive ingestion of PA-containing plants may cause severe liver damage. Because of this, the FDA asked manufacturers to stop selling oral comfrey products many years ago. Topical products are still allowed, but must clearly state on the label that they are for external use only and must be kept away from open wounds. To avoid the risks, it's best to use a comfrey that is PA-free and has been clinically studied to provide only positive benefits.

CoQ10: The Required, but Missing, Nutrient

We all need Coenzyme Q10 (CoQ10). It is present in virtually every cell in your body. But aging, medications, genetics, illness, and strenuous physical activity can greatly affect the levels of CoQ10 we have on hand. Although CoQ10 is primarily known for stopping heart disease, it is also a critical nutrient for preventing cancer, stroke, Parkinson's, migraines, and reducing the damage caused by cholesterol drugs called statin drugs.

We all make our own CoQ10 in the liver, heart, and pancreas. We can get small amounts of it from food sources, too, including; salmon, peanuts, organ meats, and whole grains. But food sources are not enough to correct low levels. One of the most important activities of CoQ10 in the body is the crucial role it plays in the way cells make energy. This cellular energy is needed for the cell to stay alive and do its job, whether it is a kidney cell or heart cell or brain cell. Healthy CoQ10 levels are associated with health and longevity.

Regardless of the ubiquitous nature of CoQ10, deficiencies are fairly common. CoQ10 levels decline with age, intensive and regular physical activity or stress, prolonged illness, and the use of drugs (statins) to lower cholesterol. In fact, one of the ways of tracking whether statin drugs are being metabolized in the liver is by noting a reduction in CoQ10 levels. One of the reasons this happens is because CoQ10 is carried by lipids—that is, it is a fat-soluble nutrient. You'll notice that most of the foods that are considered rich in

CoQ10 have some elements of natural fats or fatty acids that transport it into the body. After it is ingested, CoQ10 or ubiquinone becomes ubiquinol in the body. This is the active form, similar to the way vitamin B12 is converted from cyanocobalamin to methylcobolamin, its active form. And while CoQ10 is available as a supplement, so too is ubiquinol, often referred to as active CoQ10, or reduced CoQ10.

CoQ10 deficiencies are serious. Low CoQ10 levels are associated with cancer and migraines. They can also lead to dramatic cardiovascular and neurological health complications. Fortunately, treatment with CoQ10 can help alleviate them, too.

Stops Bad Cholesterol

CoQ10, like many nutrients, fights oxidative stress in the body. It stops the oxidation of LDL cholesterol and may boost the ability of vitamin E to stop free radical damage as well. Where cholesterol is concerned, stopping oxidation (and subsequent inflammation) is a key to stopping clogged arteries. Interestingly, a recent clinical trial added CoQ10 to the regimens of patients who were taking atorvastatin, and found that the combination was much more effective in preventing congestive heart failure than the drug used alone.

Prevents Recurrence of Heart Failure

Heart cells require a huge amount of energy production and therefore, have the highest concentration of mitochondria—considered the engine of the cell—and a great need for CoQ10. As is the case with many natural compounds, our levels of CoQ10 decline with age. But aging itself requires increased demands for CoQ10, especially in the cardiovascular system.

Additionally, as people age, muscle cells change, and the heart loses some of its ability to pump blood as vigorously. A multicenter clinical trial compared the outcomes of patients with moderate to severe heart failure over a two-year period, and how CoQ10 supplementation could improve their health. At first, at 16 weeks, they found no difference between the two groups. But after two years, the differences were quite significant. The researchers concluded that not only was CoQ10 treatment safe, but that it improved symptoms and reduced major cardiovascular events from recurring.

Controls Blood Pressure

Clinical trials of CoQ10 to treat hypertension have been positive as well. One Australian clinical study found that it improved blood pressure numbers and markers of type 2 diabetes.

A review, averaging out the results of 12 clinical studies, found that coenzyme Q10 has the potential to lower systolic blood pressure (the first number) by 17 points and diastolic blood pressure (the second number) by 10 points. For anyone with high blood pressure, or on the verge of high blood pressure, these are impressive results. And, there were no serious side effects, unlike prescription drugs.

Inhibits Parkinson's Progression

Individuals with Parkinson's disease have lower blood platelet and mitochondrial levels of CoQ10. Because of this, neurological studies of the compound have intensively focused on slowing the progression of the disease. But the results have been mixed. Earlier scientific and clinical studies showed that it slowed the progression of the disease by 44 percent, but a recent randomized study published in JAMA found no benefit for individuals with Parkinson's despite using high dosage levels.

However, researchers in Japan have recently stated that CoQ10 significantly reduced the loss of nerve signaling in the brain in scientific research. While more work needs to be done, CoQ10 should still be considered for its potential neurological benefits, and I wouldn't rule it out. Additionally, supplemental forms of CoQ10 and ubiquinol vary, and researchers are still determining which one is best absorbed and utilized by the body. It may be that the active form of CoQ10, ubiquinol, is the best choice for people with neurological diseases.

Relieves Migraines

One reason for migraine attacks may be due to the way the mitochondria—the cellular engine—functions in the brain. Working like a spark plug for this engine, CoQ10 has been used as an integrative treatment option for those who suffer from these debilitating headaches. In fact, combining it with therapeutic levels of riboflavin (vitamin B2) it appears to stabilize mitochondrial activity and relieve pain, and can reduce episodes by up to 50 percent.

Promotes Healthy Aging and Exercise Recovery

Clinical research in Spain found that healthy, older volunteers with the highest levels of CoQ10 performed the best in a series of exercises. This nutrient may be exactly what you need to keep your workouts and your physical condition at their best as you get older.

Reduces Statin Damage

One of the ways that cholesterol drugs called statins harm you is by lowering levels of an enzyme that helps synthesize CoQ10 in the body. Basically, it impedes you from making more of this nutrient. Plus, statins deplete the very lipids that carry CoQ10, so they interfere with its ability to protect the heart and arteries. The result is that they increase your risk of a heart attack, heart failure, and cause muscle pain and muscle loss due to the mitochondria being starved of necessary CoQ10. That's one of the many reasons I recommend supplementation: it can help reverse the damage brought on by statin use.

Required for Good Health

CoQ10 deficiencies are a contributing factor to many serious health concerns; cardiovascular disease, neurological conditions, breast cancer, fibromyalgia, and other degenerative diseases.

Supplementation can reduce the risk

of diabetic neuropathy, slow cognitive and motor decline, improve cholesterol balance, and reduce free-radical damage. The forms of CoQ10 vary—from the standard supplement to the active ubiquinol form—but both are highly beneficial. Supplementing with either is one of the best things you can do for your health, every day.

DOSAGE RECOMMENDATIONS

Many researchers state that the active CoQ10, ubiquinol, is at least double the strength of regular strength CoQ10 or ubiquinone. For everyday support, 50 mg of ubiquinol or 100 mg for ubiquinone should be sufficient, but for people on statins, the dose should be at least 200 mg; migraines, the dose ranges from 200–300 mg ubiquinone a day; heart disease ranges up to 400 mg daily; and the clinical study on Parkinson's disease was 1200 mg per day. Many doctors believe you can use half these amounts when using the active form.

Curcumin:
The All in One Solution

Though I am discussing some of my favorite plant medicines in this book, there is one in particular that really stands out, because of its power to make a difference in virtually every injury or disease known to humankind. If I could only take one thing to improve my health, it would be curcumin. In 45 years of studying health-related research, I have not seen anything that can match the benefits of this powerful, natural medicine.

• •

Curcumin is Powerful

Curcumin is the most potent component of turmeric, a plant that has been used in India as both a spice and medicine for centuries. Besides adding a spicy kick to Indian curry, turmeric has been used to treat conditions as varied as a toothache, gas, chest pain, and menstrual problems. Traditional practices in using turmeric for a wide variety of complaints have provided a foundation that science has built upon. By extracting curcumin from turmeric, we have an even more powerful way to treat disease. Enhancing the absorption of curcumin by blending in turmeric essential oil has resulted in a natural substance that is as potent—or even more potent—at treating disease as prescription drugs, but without the adverse effects.

Curcumin is a powerful anti-inflammatory, which is one of the reasons it works so well to treat and prevent so many diseases. That's because almost all chronic diseases—from diabetes to heart disease to arthritis to Alzheimer's disease—have something in common: unchecked, destructive inflammation. And, unlike synthetic drugs, which typically work against only a single inflammation pathway, natural curcumin reduces inflammation through its effects on multiple inflammation targets.

Curcumin is also a potent antioxidant, able to neutralize unstable, reactive free radicals. Free radicals are molecules with a missing electron that stabilize themselves by "stealing" electrons from neighboring molecules, creating another free radical in the process. This chain reaction of free radical formation is known as a free radical cascade and it can result in cellular damage (called oxidative stress) leading to inflammation and chronic disease—including cancer. Free radicals can negatively impact all body systems, including the immune system. Curcumin can stop free radical cascades without becoming unstable itself.

Beyond fighting both inflammation and oxidation, curcumin is also one of the best interventions in the world for preventing and treating cancer, making the liver healthier, reigning in insulin resistance, and helping people with depression, Alzheimer's, and other serious diseases. In fact, I can't think of a disease that would not benefit from using curcumin.

cancer is by re-awakening these "sleeping genes," turning them back on to stop cancer. This branch of science is known as epigenetics, and it may hold the answer to treating many types of cancer.

Curcumin has been shown to stop cancer initiation, promotion, and progression, meaning that it stops the changes that cause normal cells to become cancerous, stops the replication of cancerous cells (tumor formation), and stops cancerous cells from migrating to other parts of the body (known as metastasis). Published studies on curcumin's anticancer activity (so far) have found that it can suppress breast, prostate, liver, skin, oral, colon, and lung cancer. And, as an adjunct to conventional treatment, recent cell research showed that the best results for inhibiting cancer growth occurred when curcumin was used as a pretreatment *before* chemotherapy.

Curcumin has also been shown to increase the activity of cancer drugs and to decrease drug resistance in cancer cells (meaning it helps cancer drugs kill tumors more efficiently). Additionally, it

Protects Cells and Prevents Tumors

Our bodies have a natural ability to fight cancer through the activity of tumor-suppressing genes. However, aging and environmental factors can turn off or silence these genes, allowing the cancer to grow and spread unchecked. Researchers have now found that one of the ways curcumin fights

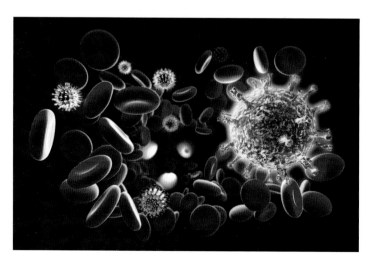

protects normal cells from the toxic effects of chemotherapy drugs and radiation treatments. Taking curcumin in combination with chemotherapy drugs may mean less of the toxic drugs are required, but the results will be better, with significantly reduced side effects. In fact, a recent clinical trial showed that a high absorption curcumin with turmeric essential oils called BCM-95 Curcumin decreased the severity of adverse effects of radiation therapy on the urinary tract in men with prostate cancer. While more research is needed, these results are so promising that you may want to discuss them with your physician if you or someone you love is involved with current or upcoming cancer treatment.

Stops Arthritis and Joint Pain

Curcumin is a remarkable botanical ingredient for anyone with osteoarthritis or rheumatoid arthritis. It protects chondrocytes, specialized cells found in joint cartilage, from being broken down by inflammatory compounds in the body. A clinical study of a combination of highly absorbable curcumin blended with turmeric essential oil and a uniquely standardized boswellia (also an excellent natural anti-inflammatory) compared it to the prescription drug celecoxib (known by the brand name, Celebrex) in the treatment of patients with osteoarthritis. The herbal combination worked better than the drug, with *no side effects*. Remarkably, 93 percent of the participants receiving the herbal combination reported reduced or no pain, compared to only 86 percent of the prescription drug group. The group receiving the special curcumin and boswellia extract were also able to walk further, and had less pain and better range of movement, all without significant adverse effects. Prescription drugs such as celecoxib are classified as non-steroidal anti-inflammatory drugs (NSAIDs) and are well known to cause adverse effects such as stomach and intestinal bleeding, ulcers, reduced kidney function, and increased blood pressure and risk of heart attack. Curcumin works just as effectively at reducing inflammation—*without* these potentially life-threatening adverse effects.

In cases of rheumatoid arthritis (RA), the body's own immune cells attack and destroy the lining of the joints (synovium). This chronic, painful, and debilitating condition is characterized by inflammation throughout the body, warm and swollen joints, and even joint destruction. Researchers examined the effects of curcumin blended with turmeric essential oil compared to the prescription drug diclofenac sodium (one brand name is Voltaren), or a combination of curcumin and diclofenac sodium in patients with rheumatoid arthritis. The group receiving the highly absorbable curcumin had the greatest reduction in joint pain and swelling with no adverse effects. In contrast, 14 percent of the participants in the drug group stopped the test because of the severity of the adverse effects they experienced.

Relieves Muscle Pain

Curcumin relieves pain from exercise and physical activity, including delayed onset muscle soreness (DOMS).

In a double-blind crossover trial, participants started taking curcumin two days before a physical workout and continued for three days after. Those taking curcumin noted moderate to large reductions in pain and slightly increased performance (due to the pain reduction). The exercises included gluteal stretches, squat jumps, and single-leg jumps, to get in a variety of controlled movements to replicate the wide range of motions that can cause pain during a workout.

Another study looked at the effects of curcumin for adult recreational cyclists. While the physical parameters were harder to judge statistically, participants in the curcumin group reported feeling "better than usual" and less stressed in the training days—two hours of endurance cycling—versus those taking placebo—even though the sessions were the same for both groups.

A four-day study featuring curcumin assessed reduction of DOMS and muscle damage in healthy adults following downhill running—a standard muscle inflammation physical test, and certainly one that can test physical limits.

The pain score in the curcumin group was 17 percent lower compared to the placebo group and there was less incidence of muscle injury in MRI. Not surprisingly, markers of inflammation and muscle damage tended to be lower in the curcumin group following exercise as well.

Fights Depression

Depression is a debilitating and difficult-to-treat disease. Approximately 30 percent of patients who take prescription drugs to relieve their depression experience no benefits, and the remaining 70 percent will have only partial improvement. Additionally, the side effects can be significant, including nausea, weight gain, dizziness, dry mouth, blurred vision, insomnia, sexual dysfunction, and more. Because curcumin has been shown to be effective at treating other brain disorders, researchers decided to explore how helpful it would be in relieving depression.

First, inflammation is known to play a major role in the development of depression so, it seems logical that the anti-inflammatory properties of curcumin would be helpful. Second, curcumin is also able to modulate the levels of brain neurotransmitters (chemical messengers—serotonin, norepinephrine, and dopamine) that influence mood, behavior, appetite, emotions, and even dreaming and memory. In experimental models of depression, curcumin has been shown to increase levels of the "feel good" neurotransmitter, serotonin, as well as relieve other symptoms of depression. In a published study comparing a special, highly absorbable curcumin with turmeric essential oil (BCM-95 Curcumin) to two prescription drugs fluoxetine (Prozac) and imipramine (Tofranil), an experimental model found the curcumin to be just as effective as the two drugs—but without the adverse side effects.

Because of these early successes, researchers developed human studies utilizing enhanced absorption curcumin with turmeric essential oil. In a clinical study, patients with major depressive disorder (MDD) showed the highest response using a combination of fluoxetine (Prozac) *and* high-absorption curcumin—a 77.8 percent response rate as measured by the Hamilton Depression Rating Scale (HAMD-17).

Interestingly, the single-therapy groups scored almost exactly the same, with fluoxetine at 64.7 percent and curcumin at 62.5 percent—numbers so close that the data is not statistically significant from one another.

Two important takeaways from this study: first, curcumin worked as well as the prescription drug fluoxetine and, second, curcumin can be an effective and

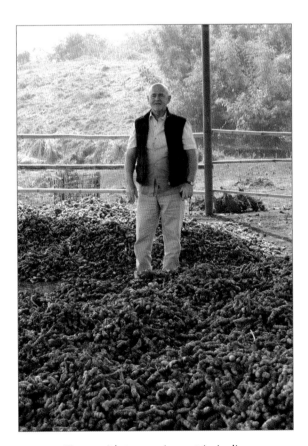

Terry with turmeric root in India.

safe treatment for patients with MDD *without* the terrible side effects that can include suicidal thoughts, interference with sexual function, and weight gain.

Another study examined two different levels of curcumin, curcumin combined with saffron or a placebo. The individuals in this trial were diagnosed with MDD, but also dealt with a subset of MDD, called "atypical depression". People with atypical depression don't respond well to conventional treatment.

The results on curcumin were impressive. The curcumin group experienced significantly reduced depression, especially the people with atypical depression. Results did not improve when saffron was added, but the curcumin-only groups were highly responsive. Many participants showed excellent improvements on the Inventory of Depressive Symptomology (IDS) scale. This means that some were likely no longer even in the category of major depression following treatment.

Preserves the Mind— Curcumin and Alzheimer's Disease

The cause of Alzheimer's disease (AD) is not entirely known. However, certain characteristic changes are found in the brains of people with this condition—accumulated clusters of a protein called beta-amyloid, and clumps of dead and dying nerve and brain cells. These clusters and clumps, called plaques and tangles, are believed to interfere with the proper transmission of messages between brain cells and lead to the death of brain cells as well. Inflammation is also believed to be involved, causing the accumulation of plaques and tangles to have even more damaging effects. Because of the known anti-inflammatory effects of curcumin, researchers are now looking at its effects in treating AD.

What they have discovered is astonishing. Not only does curcumin protect brain cells from damaging inflammation, in experimental models of Alzheimer's disease, curcumin was able to reduce beta-amyloid levels and shrink the size of accumulated plaques by over 30 percent. In fact, curcumin is more effective in inhibiting formation of beta-amyloid protein fragments than many other drugs being tested as Alzheimer's treatments. Enhanced absorption curcumin with turmeric essential oil has been clinically studied in people with Alzheimer's disease to determine the amount of beta-amyloid protein eliminated from the brain.

Other Diseases

Aside from the conditions I've covered here, I think you could recommend curcumin for virtually every disease. Curcumin can also help improve blood sugar levels and may help prevent diabetes. It improves HDL cholesterol levels, relieves the pain and bloating of IBS, and speeds skin repair and healing.

Curcumin has also shown promise in treating many other diseases and conditions, including obesity, kidney and liver disease, eye disorders, lung conditions, allergies, pancreatitis, and more. Curcumin may be able to protect against weight gain and body fat accumulation. I think curcumin is one of the most powerful natural medicines available. No matter what your health concern might be, curcumin can make a difference. That's why it is one of my favorite herbs—because it can help so many people, and even save lives.

DOSAGE RECOMMENDATIONS

I recommend BCM-95 curcumin above all others. BCM-95 is blended with turmeric essential oil for enhanced absorption and provides superior results. Many of the studies I've discussed in this chapter have shown great results with a twice daily regimen of 750 mg of curcumin enhanced with turmeric essential oil. But you could easily—and safely—go well beyond that to 3,000 mg daily (or more) for a more aggressive approach in the case of serious illnesses. And for everyday prevention in otherwise healthy adults, a dose of 375 mg of curcumin with turmeric essential oil (for a total of 375 mg) can be very useful.

TURMERIC ESSENTIAL OIL—SOURCE OF TURMERONES

As important as I think curcumin is, turmeric essential oil is an upcoming star that rightly deserves attention. Even though it hasn't gotten the press that curcumin has, the fact is, turmeric essential oil—rich in turmerones, has many of the same strengths as curcumin—and is the focus of intensive research.

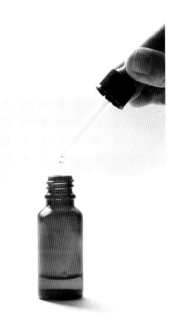

Turmerones are components of turmeric oil with anti-inflammatory and anticancer properties. It's well established that turmeric oil enhances the absorption of curcumin. More recent research has determined that turmerones make curcumin even more powerful after absorption, due to its high level of synergistic activity. Studies are showing that turmerones—especially aromatic turmerone, best known as ar-turmerone—on their own are potentially as potent as curcuminoids and have *amazing* potential to stop tumors.

Turmerones have been found to increase superoxide dismutase and glutathione level—natural antioxidants produced by the body that have incredible cell-protecting power and could practically be considered "fountains of youth" for their abilities to keep us healthy.

Aside from tumor prevention, ar-turmerone may help fight Alzheimer's and preserve cognition. A Korean study found that it suppressed beta-amyloid (responsible for the plaques and tangles in the brain that stop neural connections) and inhibited the inflammatory cytokines and pathways that cause damage to the brain.

Additionally, German research found that ar-turmerone helps regenerate brain cells—a potentially major leap for treating neurological diseases, while Belgian work has shown that turmerones may help stop epilepsy convulsions with no unwanted effects on motor function—even at what would be considered high dosage levels.

Of course, the combination of curcumin and turmeric essential oil is incredibly powerful. Laboratory work in Japan has shown that individually, curcumin and turmerones can stop colon tumor (benign adenoma) formation associated with inflammation by an impressive amount by inhibiting the activity of inflammatory enzymes. Turmerones on their own significantly inhibited tumor formation and curcumin alone also significantly inhibited tumor formation. However, combining them completely abolished tumor formation. Make no mistake—either one is strong. Together, they're unbeatable.

Devil's Claw:
For Arthritis Relief

Did you know that there is a botanical so highly respected in Europe that it accounts for 74 percent of all prescriptions written for arthritic complaints? It's devil's claw. Such noted holistic physicians as Dr. Andrew Weil and Dr. Tieraona Low Dog have recognized the herb's ability to relieve the pain and stiffness of osteoarthritis and more. Thankfully, here in the States, you can get high-quality devil's claw at your local health food store—if you understand the right questions to ask.

The Root Not the Fruit

Devil's claw—botanical name *Harpagophytum procumbens*—is native to the arid southwestern regions of Africa. The plant gets its colorful name from its fruit, which looks like a large hooked claw. However, it's the root of the plant that has been treasured by the indigenous people of Africa for centuries. Because of devils claw's potent anti-inflammatory properties, it's now used worldwide for treating arthritis. The anti-inflammatory activity of devil's claw is so powerful that its efficacy has been compared with the prescription steroid drug, cortisone.

The Devil is in the Details

Be careful about the type of devil's claw extract you choose as some are only standardized to two percent harpagosides, the key compound of the plant. Take advantage of a specialized extract standardized to 20 percent harpagosides—that way you'll get the real benefits. And, the benefits are astounding! One of the most significant pain pathways in the body is called COX-2. Devil's claw standardized to 20 percent harpagosides inhibits the COX-2 pain pathway by 31 percent. Anyone who has had to deal with the pain of joint and back woes from arthritis would be thrilled with that kind of improvement percentage. Even glucosamine and chondroitin, which received all the buzz about relief for many years, never showed this kind of effect.

In addition, devil's claw goes further than pain relief. It improves joint flexibility. One of the most important lubricants and shock absorbers your body makes is called hyaluronic acid (HA). HA is so useful medicinally that doctors sometimes inject HA into the problem joint to improve flexibility and cushioning. In a scientific study of devil's claw, researchers found that the compounds in this plant increased production of HA in the cells that line the joints by 41 percent.

Devil's claw also works because of its ability to dilate blood vessels. This dilation increases circulation of nutrient-rich blood to joints while pushing waste-laden blood away from joints. Decreased joint pain and swelling is the result.

In one study, 222 adults with mild to moderate joint disease were given devil's claw extract for eight weeks. More than half rated the devil's claw extract as "excellent" when scoring for pain, daily function, and significant improvement of stiffness. In a different clinical study, devil's claw relieved hip pain by 54 percent and knee pain by 38 percent in only eight weeks.

The bottom line? Choosing a concentrated devil's claw extract puts everything in place that is required to slow down, and possibly even reverse, the joint degeneration that is a menacing part of osteoarthritis.

Taking it One Step Better

There's no argument. Devil's claw is extremely useful for arthritis, allowing those affected by the disease to turn away from potentially harmful over-the-counter and prescription drugs. Better still, it is especially useful for issues with the back, discs, and vertebrae, because of its lubrication and cushioning power. For even more results, devil's claw can be combined with other worthy natural medicines. Proven, safe relief can be found when adding a high absorption curcumin and a specialized boswellia, to devil's claw. Now that's welcome news for the 21 million Americans dealing with arthritis.

DOSAGE RECOMMENDATION

Recommended dosage is 100 mg to 200 mg standardized to 20 percent harpagosides. Devil's claw is also highly effective in combination formulas with the anti-inflammatory herbs curcumin and boswellia.

D-Ribose:
A Special Kind of Energy

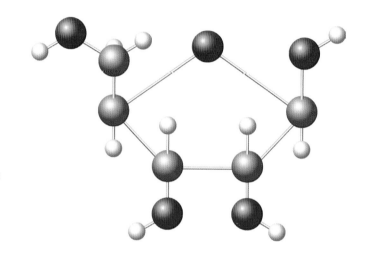

We have a molecule in our muscles called ATP (adenosine triphosphate). Depletion of ATP can result in fatigue and exhaustion. One of the key components of ATP is an unusual sugar molecule called D-ribose. It may surprise you that there are compounds in the body classified as sugar that work as building blocks, not as calories.

The Heart of the Matter

Research is showing D-ribose supplementation to be an excellent choice for skeletal muscles and perhaps our most important, vital muscle—the heart. D-ribose is also showing great promise for diseases associated with fatigue, allowing those who suffer to get back on the road to recovery.

A heart deprived of blood flow, as in a heart attack, loses the ability to pump blood efficiently. This results in a sharp drop in ATP levels. The longer the heart is deprived of oxygen-rich blood, the more it is vulnerable to damage. Getting quick recovery is crucial and D-ribose is a proven answer. In one study, people with congestive heart failure took D-ribose or a placebo for three weeks. Those taking the D-ribose showed dramatic improvement and noticed a better quality of life.

Other D-ribose Findings

Anyone dealing with fibromyalgia (FMS) and chronic fatigue syndrome (CFS) knows how debilitating fatigue can zap the energy needed for each day. One study looking at D-ribose and its effect on these syndromes found it to be well tolerated and helpful in five visual analog scale (VAS) categories: energy, sleep, mental clarity, pain intensity, and well-being. An astounding 66 percent of patients experienced significant improvement while on D-ribose. They reported an average increase in energy on the VAS of 45 percent and an average improvement in overall well-being of 30 percent.

The ABCs of ATP

Fundamentally, we need high levels of ATP to do physical activity. When levels drop, we tend to blame the fatigue and pain on many things, not understanding that the ATP levels need to be restored, and their inability to do so could be the culprit. When given the assistance of D-ribose as a key ingredient to help rejuvenate energy levels, damaged heart muscles can get back to functioning properly and providing the energy needed to exercise—something so important to heart disease prevention and recovery. Exercise enthusiasts can achieve greater goals and those who fight the battle of fibromyalgia and CFS can have new hope.

One caution: ironically, because D-ribose can lower blood glucose levels, if you are an insulin-dependent diabetic, make sure to check with your physician before taking this supplement. D-ribose provides amazing health benefits and this may be the only time you hear me speak so fondly regarding anything in the sugar family.

DOSAGE RECOMMENDATIONS

Recommended dosage of D-Ribose: 5–30 grams depending on your goals. For athletic purposes, you might use less, and for chronic fatigue/fibromyalgia, you might use more. It may also be useful to work with your healthcare professional to fully understand what dose is right for your particular health need.

Two Types of Echinacea Extracts, Widely Different Benefits

ECHINACEA Part 1: PROMOTES IMMUNE HEALTH

Echinacea (*Echinacea purpurea*) has been well-known as an immune-boosting botanical for generations. Again and again, studies find that this herbal extract reduces the length and severity of colds, and helps people get back on track much faster.

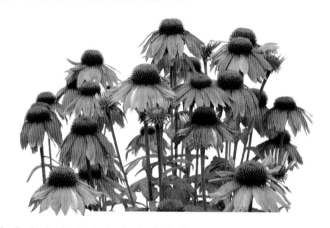

• •

Proven to Fight Cold and Flu Viruses

Compounds in echinacea stimulate the immune system. This makes echinacea especially useful when taken at the very beginning of a cold or flu, when the body needs to marshal its strength against the virus. In a recent randomized, double-blind, placebo-controlled clinical trial, an echinacea extract was tested over a 4-month period. The results were impressive: echinacea not only reduced the total number of cold episodes, but also cut the cumulative total of cold episode days within the treatment group, and the total number of occasions pain-killers were used to relieve other symptoms. It was also shown to inhibit colds and prevent viral infections.

Another review of complementary treatments for colds and flu found that *Echinacea purpurea* was consistently the most effective choice. The researchers found that symptom severity was reduced in four out of six trials, and in the four trials that measured the duration of cold symptoms, the reduction was significant—in some cases by three or four days!

I am often asked if it is safe to use echinacea if you have an autoimmune disease. The theoretical concern is that use of an herb that improves or "boosts" the immune system might fuel an increase in over-activity that, in turn, may exacerbate an auto-immune condition like lupus, or rheumatoid arthritis. It has been my experience that this is not true, but this idea has persisted as a myth. It turns out that the part of the immune system that echinacea affects is not the same part of the immune system that is malfunctioning in an autoimmune disease. There have been a few studies and review articles on this topic, including a study of people with an autoimmune disease whose use of echinacea actually improved the disease (idiopathic autoimmune uveitis). When echinacea was first promoted in Germany in the late 1930s, there was no data available to know whether or not echinacea would affect autoimmunity, so the experts decided to err on the side of caution. They did not recommend its use for people with an autoimmune condition. As science has progressed and more is known, that thinking has changed. Several world experts on echinacea have confirmed to me that this early theory has no scientific basis.

DOSAGE RECOMMENDATIONS

When supplementing with *Echinacea purpurea* for immune reasons, it's best to take at least 150–160 mg three times daily.

ECHINACEA Part 2: RELIEVES ANXIETY (*WHO KNEW?!*)

It may surprise you to learn that echinacea has a secret. There is a unique compound of echinacea, a type of echinacoside that has profound anti-anxiety activity when it is extracted as a purified extract. The species richest in this compound is *Echinacea angustifolia.* It's important to note that this is *not* the same kind of echinacea extract that you'd use for cold and flu prevention and treatment. Instead, Hungarian researchers working extensively with this unique compound have found it effective for generalized anxiety disorder (GAD) and for use in stressful situations.

Approximately 40 million Americans age 18 and older have some form of anxiety disorder, which makes a safe, natural treatment like this one extremely relevant. Anxiety affects everything we do. It makes us feel overwhelmed, destroys our ability to rest and sleep, harms our immunity, and stops us from experiencing joy. Unfortunately, prescription drugs for anxiety often cause serious side effects. Thankfully, this specialized, clinically tested botanical calms the nervousness and fears that take a toll on mental and physical health. It also matches the symptom relief of prescription anti-anxiety medications, but without serious side effects.

In one study, seven types of echinacea extracts were compared to the prescription anti-anxiety drug, chlordiazepoxide (also known by the brand name Librium®). Only one echinacea preparation—*Echinacea angustifolia*—demonstrated a robust ability to reduce anxiety in a wide dosage range comparable to the prescription drug. This extract not only met the drug's anti-anxiety effects, it exceeded them. It also didn't cause any drowsiness—a common side effect of prescription drugs for anxiety. Aside from drowsiness and lethargy, the other adverse effects for chlordiazepoxide include confusion, edema, nausea, constipation, menstrual abnormalities, jaundice, altered libido, involuntary movements, and controlled substance dependence/addiction.

And the potentially serious adverse effects for this special echinacea preparation? None.

Fast-Acting, Dramatic Results

In one published human clinical trial, the special purified extract of *Echinacea angustifolia* was tested with individuals experiencing increased anxiety and tension. After just one day, the participants noticed a significant reduction in stress and anxiety, with an even greater reduction in just seven days.

Another study focused on individuals who were diagnosed with generalized anxiety disorder (GAD) according to DSM-IV (Diagnostics and Statistical Manual of Mental Disorders) criteria. The study started with a screening phase, followed by six weeks of double-blind treatment. Participants received either 40 mg of the special *Echinacea angustifolia* extract or placebo tablets twice daily. Between visits one and six during the treatment period, the number of severely anxious patients (HADS-A scores larger than 11) decreased from 11 to zero in the echinacea group. This specialized echinacea preparation significantly reduced anxiety in GAD patients, with a full effect within about 21 days.

Powerful Relief of Anxiety

This specialized extract showed dramatic results with 40 mg taken twice daily. If you're suffering from considerable anxiety and stress, I recommend taking that level for at least one week. As your anxiety subsides, and you feel calmer; you can reduce the dosage to just 20 mg twice daily, and make it part of your regular regimen.

This is simply one of the best natural products I've seen for anxiety and stress. It has no serious side effects, and it can be used long term, combined with other medicines. Even children age four and up with anxiety can take between 20 and 40 mg daily. If you only deal with occasional bouts of anxiety, try 20 mg before a stressful event, such as public speaking, a presentation, or air travel. You'll feel calmer, less nervous, and more in control.

DOSAGE RECOMMENDATIONS

If you struggle with stress, anxiety, nervous tension, and restless sleep, take 20–40 mg of standardized *Echinacea angustifolia* EP107 extract two times daily. An additional dose can be added at bedtime if needed.

Elderberry:
A Powerhouse for Immunity

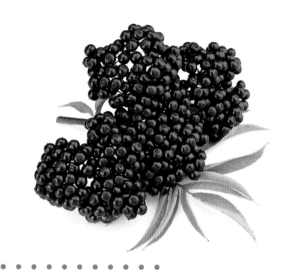

Elderberry is a powerful, botanical ingredient that has the proven ability to disrupt viruses and restore the body's capacity to fight them off without the use of prescription medication. In today's fast-paced world—elderberry is a welcome solution!

A Multi-Purpose Berry

Elderberry (*Sambucus nigra*) comes from white flowers on a bushy tree that's part of the honeysuckle family. The flowers turn into berry clusters in late summer to early fall. In this usage, it is what was used for centuries. Hippocrates referred to the elderberry bush as his "medicine chest" as early as 400 BC. Native Americans also recognized the value of the berry. They used many aspects of the plant for tools and arrows as well as medicinally for everything from colds and flu to arthritis relief, upset stomach, and reducing congestion. In 1899, an American sailor found that the wine he was drinking, which had added elderberries for color, helped with his arthritis pain. This discovery set off a series of circumstances that led to medical use and continued studies of the elderberry.

Today we know that elderberries have exceptional antiviral and anti-inflammatory properties with antioxidant capabilities to help prevent cell damage. Elderberries have more flavonol content than blackberries, blueberries, cranberries, and goji berries. They are a good source of fiber and vitamin A and contain or deliver an amazing 87 percent of the infection-fighting vitamin C, providing more than any other plant beside rosehips and black currants. Other prominent ingredients in elderberries include iron, potassium, vitamin B6, and lots of beta-carotene.

Studied and Proven

Elderberry is one of the most clinically studied herbs for fighting colds and the flu. For anyone who travels or has a lot of contact with people, elderberry saves the day. An Australian clinical trial found that taking a standardized extract of elderberry while traveling cut the risk of colds and flu in half. The type of elderberry extract I recommend, the Haschberg variety is a freeze-dried ingredient. This is the type used in the Australian trial. It removes the water content without damaging the beneficial compounds in the berry. In addition, this type of freeze-dried extract retains the highest levels of antioxidants, anthocyanins, and other components and has the longest shelf life of any drying process.

Another study suggested that elderberry extract could shorten flu duration by up to three days. The extract worked so well that researchers compared it with the prescription medication most commonly prescribed for the flu. If you feel a cold or flu coming on, reach for elderberry. It's a good idea to use a formula that combines other immune boosters like vitamin A, vitamin C, vitamin D, magnesium, calcium lactate, and zinc for a strong defense against these viruses.

There is also ongoing research on elderberry and its ability to stimulate the body's immune system for patients dealing with diseases like cancer and AIDS and for viral illnesses like shingles.

DOSAGE RECOMMENDATIONS

A good standard dosage is 300 mg of elderberry in one daily tablet. You can use this dosage every day for long-term protection. If you actually have a viral illness, like a cold or the flu, increase the elderberry or a formula with elderberry to three to six times daily, for up to seven days. You should feel much better by then and can return to your once daily dosage.

Eleuthero: Adaptation Is the Key to Good Health

If you find yourself feeling overwhelmed, there are many ways of getting back on track. Discovering eleuthero (*Eleutherococcus senticosus*)—formerly known as "Siberian ginseng"—may be one of the best. It helps you adapt to stressful times and reenergize when you need it. This herb has been cherished for centuries. "I would rather have a handful of Wucha (Eleuthero) than a cartload of gold and jewels," wrote the famous Chinese herbalist Li Shi-Chen, in his 1596 treatise on herbal medicine *Ben Cao Gang Mu*.

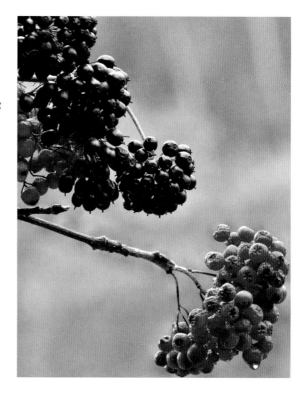

• •

In fact, adapting is exactly what this botanical—considered a premier *adaptogen*—is suited for. Adaptogens provide us with exactly the appropriate support we need, exactly when we need it. If you need more physical stamina and endurance, eleuthero can provide the energy boost. If you need more mental focus, it bolsters that, too.

Eleuthero is native to far eastern Russia, Northern Korea, China, and Japan.

Intensive study and traditional use has shown that it is an essential herb for mental and physical endurance and much more.

For that reason, it isn't surprising that eleuthero is associated with improved mental health, increased physical endurance, stronger immune health, and reduced levels of cortisol—the "fight or flight" hormone that can cause a spiral of stress to get worse.

Eleuthero Research

In one double-blind study, participants age 65 and older used the herb or a placebo for a total of eight weeks. Surveys taken by the participants showed that the eleuthero group was already noting better mental health and more comfort in social situations at just four weeks into the study.

Another double-blind study examined the cardiovascular response to stress and eleuthero benefits. The eleuthero group showed a 40 percent reduction in their heart rate when responding to a standard clinical stress test compared to the placebo group. And while the research is still ongoing, studies also point to eleuthero as being an excellent choice to help you accomplish tasks better and with less confusion, if you're running short on sleep. Additionally, in combination with rhodiola and schisandra (two other potent adaptogens) eleuthero may boost neurological factors in individuals with chronic anxiety.

Exercise can be extremely beneficial if you're looking for ways to deal with stress and have more energy. Exercise improves energy and energy makes it more likely you'll be active. It has also been shown in studies that you have a better attitude toward life in general if you're able to get physical activity on a regular basis. Eleuthero can help with this, too—it has been shown to enhance physical endurance and help the cardiovascular system keep the pace.

The key compounds from eleuthero that are responsible for these remarkable abilities are called "eleutherosides" and are standardized from the root of the plant. You should make sure that the product you select is standardized for eleutheroside content. That way you'll know you're getting the compound that shows results. As part of a combination of synergistic adaptogens, you probably won't need quite as much. But whether you call this adaptogenic herb "Siberian ginseng" or more properly "eleuthero," it can boost your energy levels, improve your response to stressful situations, and bolster your workouts all at the same time. It is one of my favorite herbs, and it will help you adapt to whatever life sends your way.

DOSAGE RECOMMENDATIONS

If you're taking this botanical as a single ingredient, I think that 300–400 mg (two or three times daily) of the extract standardized to eleutherosides is sufficient.

Eucalyptus:
A Gift from Australia

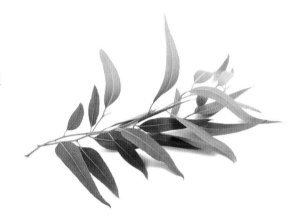

Native to Australia, eucalyptus is best known as the preferred food of koala bears and for its distinctive pungent aroma. But its true value lies in the essential oil's ability to ease inflammation, relieve congestion, and battle a wide range of bacteria.

• •

There are several varieties of eucalyptus used to make the essential oil, but I recommend the oil of *Eucalyptus radiate.* This particular variety contains 65 to 70 percent 1,8 cineole, as well as alpha-pinene and limonene—all compounds with strong anti-inflammatory, decongestant, and anti-bacterial abilities.

Research also suggests that eucalyptus essential oil boasts analgesic, or pain-relieving, properties. One study in the *American Journal of Physical Medicine and Rehabilitation* found that the essential oil provided pain relief and acted as a passive form of warm-up for athletes who applied it topically.

Breathe Easy

Thanks to its powerful scent, just one whiff of eucalyptus oil can instantly clear sinus passages, making it exceptional for treating head colds, allergies, and sinusitis. Used in capsule form, this natural oil has the unique ability to thin mucus so it can drain from the body more easily. It also stimulates cilia activity in the lungs and sinuses. Cilia are tiny projections that constantly sweep debris out of the lungs and sinus passages for elimination. And because eucalyptus contains both antibacterial and antiviral properties, it's also an excellent treatment for sinus infections.

In addition to the ability to fight viruses, the 1,8 cineole compound in eucalyptus is proving to be a safe and effective replacement for steroid medications in the treatment of chronic asthma. A study conducted at the Medical Outpatient Clinic at Bonn University Hospital in Germany showed the effectiveness of the oral compound for asthma patients. The results conveyed that 12 of the 16 patients in the cineole group (versus 4 of the 16 patients in the placebo group) were able to reduce their use of conventional steroid anti-inflammatory medicine.

Kick Candida

Eucalyptus is also effective in combatting yeast infections, which are caused by the overgrowth of common fungus known as *Candida albicans.* While yeast symptoms vary widely and can often seem unrelated, one common thread is the systemic inflammation that yeast causes in the body. This inflammation can cause swelling in the mouth, vaginal irritation, and IBS symptoms. This inflammation forces the body to spend its energy fighting candida overgrowth instead of reducing the inflammation caused by the fungus.

In addition to relieving inflammation, eucalyptus oil has been found to have direct antifungal effects against a variety of fungal species, including *Aspergillus fumigatus, Cryptococcus neoformans* (another potentially dangerous yeast that can cause lung infections and fungal meningitis) and of course, *candida albicans.*

DOSAGE RECOMMENDATIONS

When choosing a eucalyptus supplement, remember to look for one that contains 65 to 70 percent 1,8 cineole. An effective dose of eucalyptus is 125 mg, up to six times daily. Also, the best delivery system for any essential oil is in a base of extra virgin olive oil. Try to avoid products that use canola or other unhealthy oils.

Unique Fiber Effective for Weight Loss

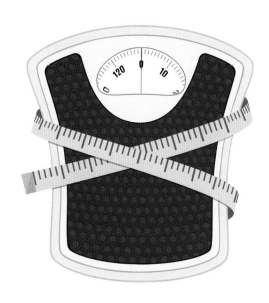

By now, I think everyone is pretty much aware that fiber is a key component of weight loss. There are a few reasons for this. First, fiber fills you up. The fact that it touches on multiple points within the digestive system essentially stops the sensation of hunger. That's why you'll see fiber-rich foods recommended for anyone who is trying to lose weight. First, many fiber-rich fruits and vegetables (I would skip grains) are typically full of other healthy compounds, so they're great for many reasons. Secondly, with enough of them in your daily regimen, you're simply not going to have that "empty" feeling that signals you to eat more.

Aside from that very valuable reason, fiber moves toxins out of the body, absorbs fat, and balances blood sugar levels, too. So you get a combined effect of feeling less hungry and having fewer highs and lows in your blood sugar levels, which would otherwise trigger another bout of eating.

• •

Special, Clinically Studied Fiber

I absolutely think you should add nutrient-and-fiber-rich fruits and vegetables to your plan for weight loss. Along with that, I'd recommend a clinically studied form of chitosan from plant fiber.

Chitosan is derived from chitin, a structural ingredient found in shellfish or the cell walls of the mushroom family.

However, chitosan derived from shellfish can use pretty harsh processing techniques and turn people off due to dietary sensitivities or practices. However, chitosan from a plant-based source provides all the benefits of a supplemental form of fiber with none of the processing or sourcing concerns.

In just 3 months, with no dietary restrictions (although I think diet is *extremely* important) people lost up to 7 times the weight of those in the placebo group, who on average *gained* half of a pound.

Weight Loss and Better Blood Sugar

Overall, people in the fiber group saw significantly lower BMI, body fat, visceral fat (fat accumulated around organs in the torso, a typically dangerous type), and waist, hip, and upper abdominal circumference. Another real plus is that those in the fiber group saw lower A1C levels, too—the average levels of blood sugar over time, and a way to gauge diabetes.

Diabetes and being overweight are often conditions that happen in tandem. Fiber in general is a good way to fight both, and I encourage anyone with blood sugar concerns or someone who wants to lose weight to add this fiber to their daily regimen. The best results happen when you make a point of taking this fiber source about 15 minutes to one hour before a meal. That may seem tough to remember sometimes, but even setting a reminder on your phone or jotting a note on your calendar can prompt you to take the supplement in advance of your meals and help you achieve your healthy goals.

DOSAGE RECOMMENDATIONS

Take 500–1,000 mg of fiber about 20 to 30 minutes before meals. For weight loss benefits, use two to three times daily.

Ginger: A Spicy Solution

Looking inside your spice cabinet, you probably have some ginger that you use in baking and cooking. Even though ginger is one of the world's ten favorite spices, it offers us much more than an additive to baked goods. With an ability to relieve pain, settle the stomach, act as an excellent anti-inflammatory and more, it's time to take a new look at an ancient yet timely herb you might be taking for granted—ginger.

A Spice with a Price

Ginger (*Zingiber officinale*) comes from the same family as cardamom and turmeric. Because it was widely cultivated and secretly traded, many believe it originated in southern China, although not all scholars agree. Lucrative ginger trades had an enormous impact on economic history, much like oil and water affect our economy today. It was revered for its medicinal value and the ability to preserve food.

Ginger as Medicine

It's the oil derived from the underground rhizome of the ginger plant, the bulbous part just above the roots that is valued as a natural medicine. The primary compounds found in the ginger oil are the pungent gingerols and shogaols that account for the majority of the health benefits. These compounds interrupt inflammatory triggers that can cause the development, growth, and spread of tumors and the cycle of cancer development.

One example of ginger's power is the ability to treat glioblastoma, an aggressive form of brain cancer. This type of cancer spreads quickly and can often become resistant to chemotherapy. In a cell study, gingerol was combined with a type of therapy to fight this particular cancer. The results suggested chemoresistance to the therapy would be less likely because of the ginger. In another ginger/chemotherapy related study assessing ginger's ability to reduce nausea, 576 cancer patients undergoing chemotherapy were given ginger or a placebo. The results showed a reduction in acute nausea for the ginger group, and less use of an anti-nausea drug compared to the placebo group.

Alone and Together

Researchers are finding out more and more about all that ginger oil offers. It's a long list including an effect on cognitive function, as an antidepressant, for heart disease, cholesterol, blood pressure, as an anti-inflammatory, for digestion and all types of nausea, liver disease, chronic pain and osteoarthritis, osteoporosis, cancer, diabetes, and metabolic syndrome to name a few.

Combining ginger with turmeric essential oil has also been found to provide astounding clinical benefits. Turmerones are the main component of turmeric essential oil. Combining it with ginger oil standardized for gingerols and shogaols through a supercritical CO_2 extraction is a perfect combination for fighting DNA-damaging oxidative stress, dealing with inflammation, and optimizing the cell's protective abilities. To protect your cells from damage and reduce chronic inflammation, I recommend taking ginger oil standardized to a minimum of 25 percent gingerols and shogaols, as well as turmeric oil standardized to a minimum of 60 percent turmerones, daily.

I hope that this glimpse at ginger as a natural medicine will encourage you to explore the many ways it goes beyond a popular spice to being the answer for a multitude of today's health issues.

DOSAGE RECOMMENDATIONS

Dosages vary widely on ginger, but anywhere from 150–750 mg daily of a standardized ginger can be very beneficial. The ginger you choose should be standardized to contain at least 25% total gingerols and shogaols.

Ginkgo: A Powerful Brain Booster

Native to China, *Ginkgo biloba* is a living fossil, the last surviving member of a tree family from over 200 million years ago. It has remained virtually unchanged since the age of the dinosaurs. The trees are large—reaching up to 120 feet high—and often live for well over 1,000 years. Ginkgo trees are mighty and lasting, and they provide one of the most popular herbal supplements in the world.

There are more than 40 components in ginkgo, but according to scientists, only two are believed to contribute to gingko's health benefits: flavonoids and terpenoids. Both of these contain powerful antioxidant properties proven to offer an array of nutritional benefits for brain, heart, and more.

• • • • • • • • • • • • • • • • • • • •

Improving Brain Health

A multitude of studies have shown that ginkgo is effective for improving both cognition and memory. It works by boosting blood flow to the brain, destroying free radicals, and protecting brain cells from premature death.

Research specifically shows that ginkgo has a positive effect on memory and thinking for people with Alzheimer's disease or vascular dementia. It is believed that it may help people who have Alzheimer disease improve their ability to think, learn, and remember. The herb may also help to improve social behavior and the ability to perform daily tasks.

For those who do not have Alzheimer's disease, ginkgo may help protect against age-related mental decline. There is also research suggesting its usefulness for the treatment of children with Attention Deficit Hyperactivity Disorder, or ADHD.

Lessening Stroke Damage

Researchers also continue to study ginkgo's role in the prevention and treatment of stroke. It's believed that by preventing blood clots from developing and increasing the blood flow to the brain, the herb may prevent strokes from occurring. It's also believed that the herb inhibits free-radical damage of brain cells after a stroke.

Additional Benefits

Ginkgo biloba has also been studied for its efficacy in the treatment of other health conditions including Raynaud's phenomenon, premenstrual syndrome, glaucoma, multiple sclerosis, anxiety, and more. If you're interested in taking a ginkgo supplement, you'll want to look for one that is standardized to contain 24 percent flavone glycosides and 6 percent terpene lactones.

DOSAGE RECOMMENDATIONS

Studies regarding ginkgo biloba have used anywhere from 120–600 mg daily. It's a good idea to start at a lower dose until you find what works best for you.

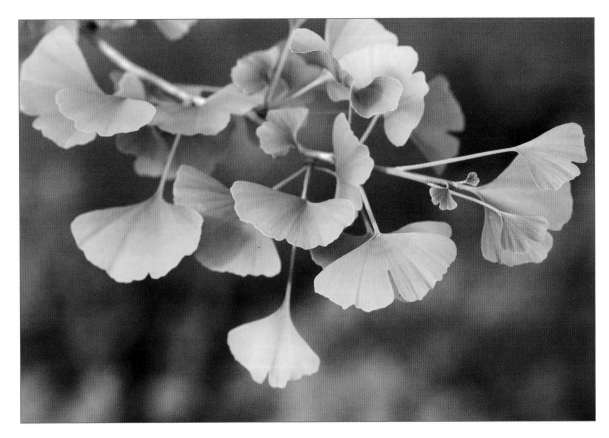

Ginseng: The Divine Plant

Ginseng, like many of the herbs I discuss in this book, has been long recommended for virtually every health condition for thousands of years, originally in traditional Chinese, Korean, and Japanese medical practice. Ginseng is called "The Divine Plant" because of its extraordinary value, and is considered one of the most precious herbal medicines in the Chinese Pharmacopeia. The dried root of the plant provides many powerful compounds, first among them, triterpene saponins called *ginsenosides* that make the herb extremely beneficial for energy, focus, and longevity.

• • • • • • • • • • • • • • • • • • • •

Much like other adaptogens, ginseng has yielded remarkable results for a wide spectrum of conditions, including keeping your focus—even after glucose consumption (maybe a cure for post-lunch slumps), cancer-related fatigue, immune resistance, and serious cognitive symptoms.

For instance, if you deal with a drop in concentration and start to feel sleepy after meals, my first advice would be to drop the carbohydrates and see if that makes a difference. My second would be to try adding ginseng to your afternoon regimen. It doesn't contain caffeine, so if you're sensitive to that, and concerned about losing sleep, don't worry.

Powerful Benefits

In a clinical test, young adult volunteers fasted overnight, and then were given a 10-minute "cognitive demand" test the following morning for a baseline read on how well everyone could perform. Then they either consumed ginseng or a placebo. Half an hour later, they were given a glucose drink or a placebo beverage.

After thirty minutes went by, the volunteers completed six "cognitive demand" tests in a row. The ginseng and glucose group scored better on math portions of the test and felt less fatigue in the latter tests. It also seemed that ginseng reduced overall glucose levels in those who had not received the additional glucose. The researchers didn't feel that the ginseng and glucose were necessarily showing synergistic effects, but rather that the ginseng would probably moderate glucose levels.

These results were a follow up on earlier research that showed that ginseng could overcome glucose loads when cognitive focus was needed—similar batteries of tests and similar results. Ginseng improved the test performance and the subjective feelings of fatigue after sustained mental workouts. The study authors concluded that one of the reasons for this was the herb's ability to deal with blood sugar levels.

And if you're not always regular with your regimen, but still want the effects of ginseng, you're in luck: even short-term use (in this case, 400 mg a day) can be enough to improve calm and cognitive ability.

Boost Performance

Beyond glucose regulation, ginseng is considered by some to be a special class of adaptogen—something called an "acto-protector." In this case, ginseng boosts your mental and physical performance without increasing oxygen consumption in the body. In other words, you get more mileage with the same amount of fuel. If you have a daily workout, ginseng may be an excellent addition.

Ginseng may also help you re-energize if you deal with symptoms of chronic daily fatigue. Researchers observed that it increased levels of glutathione—the body's natural antioxidant and "fountain of youth

and energy" and reduced free radical stresses that can zap our natural vitality.

At MD Anderson Cancer Center, ginseng was shown to relieve cancer-related fatigue and improve appetite and better sleep at night in 87 percent of the patients in the study. These are all primary issues during treatment, so ginseng may be on the cusp of making life much better for more people.

Safe and Effective

One of the reasons that researchers can trust ginseng is that it is incredibly safe. Ginseng doesn't interfere with drugs or your liver's ability to detoxify, and may even be a potential therapeutic herb to help people with non-alcoholic fatty liver disease overcome fatigue brought about by the condition.

The risk of infections following surgery is a great threat, especially since antibiotics have been overused and are often ineffective. Research with Korean ginseng shows that it protects host cells against *pneumococcal sepsis*—a potential cause of meningitis, and responsible for over half of post-operative hospital deaths. Ginseng also stops viruses from replicating as well and enhances the strength of cells.

Of course, ginseng is well regarded and known for enhancing sexual performance and satisfaction for men *and* women— another example of its adaptogenic abilities.

Overall, as a restorative, protective, and energizing herb, I think ginseng is one of the best. It has an uncanny ability to adapt to your needs, and makes an excellent addition to a daily regimen.

DOSAGE RECOMMENDATIONS

Depending on the condition, dosage levels for ginseng can vary: positive results for focus and attention have been seen at 100–200 mg per day and relief for cancer-related fatigue has been found for 800 mg per day. I think you could easily start at 200 mg and see how well it works for your energy levels. For those with fatigue issues, a minimum of four percent extract of up to 400 mg was used, but the results differed little from the group at the 1,000 mg level, so extremely high doses are usually not necessary.

NORTH AMERICAN VS. ASIAN GINSENG—WHAT'S THE DIFFERENCE?

There is more than one ginseng.

I live in Green Bay, Wisconsin, and in the northern part of our state, ginseng thrives in the wild and is also cultivated. The ginseng in Wisconsin and throughout North America is considered a different species—*Panax quinquefolius*—but exhibits many of the same characteristics when it's applied clinically.

In fact, there has been some fascinating research showing that North American ginseng can protect the cardiovascular system and Wisconsin ginseng has been shown to reduce cancer-related fatigue, much like *Panax ginseng* from Asia.

I would suggest that if you're interested in ginseng, that you try both and see which one works best for you. They are both incredibly beneficial herbs that can enhance your life.

Glutathione: The Longevity Key

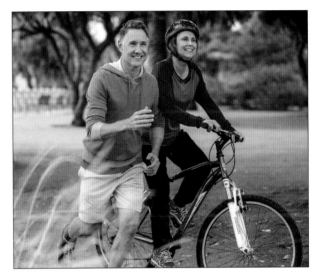

When we hear the word *antioxidant*, there are many foods and herbs that come to mind. Antioxidants are so crucial for life that our body makes two special ones to ensure our survival: superoxide dismutase, and the incredibly important glutathione. Glutathione is so important that it is often referred to as the "mother of antioxidants."

Protects Against Factors that Accelerate Aging

Glutathione is a combination of three amino acids: cysteine, glycine, and glutamate. With the ability to neutralize substances like free radicals, metabolic waste, heavy metals, toxins, and other harmful substances, glutathione truly is key to a vibrant life. Every cell in the body is capable of making glutathione, and glutathione is also made by the liver and released into the bloodstream. Before we were born, our bodies were producing this important substance to facilitate proper development. Disruptions in glutathione production can lead to life-threatening or chronic illnesses.

Conversely, people who are naturally good at making glutathione tend to live longer-than-normal lifespans. Healthy people over 100 years of age tend to have significantly higher levels of glutathione production than the general population.

There are two forms of glutathione that are found in our body at any given time: the active form (reduced glutathione) and the inactive form (oxidized glutathione). Once active glutathione has neutralized a toxic substance it changes into the inactive form. The inactive glutathione can be recycled back into active glutathione or broken down and eliminated from the body. In healthy adults, there should be around 90 percent of the body's glutathione supply that is in the active form and only 10 percent that is in the inactive form. In a 2009 scientific study, researchers found that children who have autism only have about 60 percent of their glutathione in the active form and 40% in the inactive form. The ratio between active to inactive glutathione is an important indicator of overall health.

Research and Results

Researchers have also explored glutathione's effects on Parkinson's disease, cancer, Lyme disease, Alzheimer's disease, heart disease, rheumatoid arthritis, and countless others. Glutathione is able to protect cells from certain kinds of damage, which can lead to chronically high levels of inflammation. And it has recently been discovered that chronic inflammation lies at the root cause of almost every disease and illness. Scientific studies on glutathione have found it is very useful for any disease with underlying oxidative stress and inflammation, but especially for the diseases that affect the neurological system.

One particular study involving people with Parkinson's disease demonstrated that glutathione treatment could drastically reduce their symptoms. The patients were given intravenous (IV) glutathione for thirty days. At the end of the study, there was a 42 percent reduction in symptoms and the effects lasted for more than two months after the glutathione treatment was concluded. More research needs to be done, but I think this is a very important supplement to consider in Parkinson's disease.

Not All Forms Work

Most of the scientific studies use IV glutathione because it keeps glutathione in the active form. Other supplemental forms of glutathione that are swallowed, even those that are enteric-coated, become oxidized during the digestive process. This means that supplemental glutathione can actually do harm in the body because it is delivering the wrong form of glutathione.

The form of glutathione I prefer has been scientifically shown to improve the ratio of active (favorable) vs inactive (unfavorable) glutathione. This particular form of glutathione comes from France and is designed to be absorbed under the tongue (sublingual). The glutathione is kept in the active form with the addition of natural polyphenols from pomegranate. In a three week study using this patented form of sublingual glutathione, it improved the ratio of active to inactive glutathione 230 percent better than unprotected glutathione and 65 percent better than N-acetylcysteine (a precursor to glutathione). The results are incredibly impressive considering the study only lasted three weeks. A side benefit of increased glutathione levels included a significant increase in vitamin C and E levels, because glutathione keeps these valuable vitamins active in the body longer.

Many of us go out of our way to eat a healthy diet that contains organic fruits, vegetables, clean protein, and good fats. The addition of glutathione to your routine can help the antioxidants in your diet have even more potent benefits.

Glutathione is a nutrient you cannot get from your diet. The proven effective forms for delivering active glutathione are either IV or sublingual (under the tongue). However, it is important to look for a glutathione that is clinically proven to improve active glutathione levels and also the ratio of active to inactive glutathione.

DOSAGE RECOMMENDATIONS

For maintenance of good health, 150 mg of slow-melt gluta-thione is sufficient for most people. These tablets are designed to melt slowly in the mouth, preferably under the tongue. To address more serious health concerns, anywhere from 300–600 mg of slow-melt glutathione per day may be necessary.

THE PROBLEM WITH SOME PAIN DRUGS

Glutathione levels decrease with age, poor nutrition, toxins and pollution, infections and diseases, trauma, and certain drugs, especially acetaminophen. When it comes to main-taining healthy levels of glutathione in the body, limiting or avoiding any drugs with acetaminophen is absolutely necessary. While every cell can produce glutathione, the majority of this production occurs in the liver. A healthy liver is necessary to maintain proper glutathione production and recycling in the body.

Acetaminophen is metabolized by the liver and can destroy many liver cells during this process. In fact, acetaminophen toxicity is the number one cause of acute liver failure in the United States. Because many common prescription and over-the-counter medications contain acetaminophen, it can be easy to consume too much of this potentially harmful substance. Very high doses of acetaminophen can reduce glutathione levels by over 80 percent, which can lead to life-threatening complications.

To maintain healthy levels of glutathione, I encourage you to seek out safer aceta-minophen alternatives whenever possible. If you are using acetaminophen for pain management, try a combination of curcumin, boswellia, DLPA, and nattokinase instead.

Grape Seed Extract: Good Things Come in Small Packages

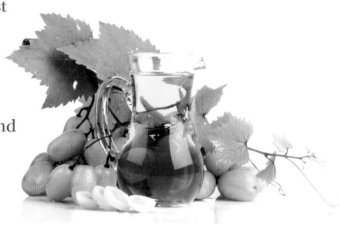

Grape seed extract is one of the most powerful natural medicines available. This amazing botanical has the ability to prevent heart disease, stop diabetes and prevent weight gain, slow the progression of brain disease, and even kill cancer cells. It is truly one of nature's "do everything" ingredients. I think everyone would benefit from including grape seed extract in their daily health regimen.

Not All Grape Seed Extract Is Created Equal

When looking for an effective grape seed extract, size matters. Oligomeric proanthocyanidin complexes (OPCs) are compounds found in grape seeds that have great protective value, but to be beneficial, they need to be small. Grape seed extract that contains only small OPCs is the most easily absorbed by the body and can do wonders for your health.

Tannins are OPCs too, but are too big to be absorbed by the body. Unfortunately, many grape seed extracts are simply all tannins. Technically, tannins and OPCs are both proanthocyanidins. But tannins have little value because they cannot be absorbed. The best grape seed products are tannin free. Small OPCs are water soluble and highly bioavailable, and that's what will make the difference for your health. The grape seed extract I recommend is a French variety called VX1. VX1 is tannin-free, and has unique specifications that make it highly absorbable.

Protects Cardiovascular Health

Grape seed extract reduces high blood pressure, protects the blood vessel walls from free radical damage, and prevents the dangerous oxidation of LDL cholesterol—one of the first steps on the road to a heart attack or stroke.

In an Italian clinical study, individuals with pre- or mild-hypertension were divided into three groups, two with grape seed extract at lower and higher dosages, and one with a diet and exercise intervention only, serving as a control group. At the end of the four-month trial, both grape seed extract groups saw an improvement in blood pressure, although those at the higher dosage noticed more dramatic effects. In fact, blood pressure numbers returned to normal in 93 percent of those in the higher dosage group.

I do not think there is much benefit in reducing cholesterol, as it is such an important compound in the body. However, cholesterol balance can be important—the ratio of HDL to LDL cholesterol and triglycerides, too. A clinical study compared the results of individuals with mildly high cholesterol taking a grape seed extract versus a placebo for eight weeks. Lipid profiles and oxidized LDL (bad) cholesterol were improved in those taking grape seed extract.

Other scientific studies have found similar results: grape seed extract helps prevent blood clots from forming without thinning the blood, lowers blood pressure, and shields blood vessels and arteries from free radical damage.

Stops Diabetes and Obesity

As the number of people dealing with type 2 diabetes grows, researchers will continue to find natural answers that work with the body to normalize blood sugar levels and heal the damage to blood vessels and nerves. A pilot clinical study in Thailand found that grape seed extract reduced blood sugar levels after a high-carbohydrate meal. The OPCs in grape seed can help stop the sugar spikes that affect insulin levels and possibly lead to diabetes.

Laboratory studies also show that grape seed extract can protect against damage caused by diabetes, including diabetic neuropathy and the risk of cardiovascular complications, like heart disease. Other laboratory work found that an exercise regimen combined with grape seed extract reduced triglycerides, improved total cholesterol ratios, aided weight loss, and lowered systolic blood pressure.

Slows Alzheimer's Progression and Promotes Focus

Grape seed OPCs also have strong anti-oxidant and anti-inflammatory activity, which makes them beneficial for brain health. Studies have shown that grape seed protects the delicate circuitry of the brain, which is of major concern for Alzheimer's patients. For example, an Indian study found that grape seed proanthocyanidins reduce the effects of oxidative stress in the aging brain and consider it a neuroprotectant to prevent cognitive loss.

Prevent Cancer and Tumor Growth

Another exciting benefit of grape seed extract is its extraordinary ability to fight cancer cells and prevent tumor proliferation.

One study found that a tannin-free French grape seed extract standardized to only small-sized OPCs suppressed colorectal cancer cells in a variety of ways. It inhibited the growth of tumors, stopped the cycle of cancer cell signaling, and induced apoptosis—the death of cancer cells. But perhaps even more importantly, it also killed cancer stem cells.

This is an amazing breakthrough because even though conventional chemotherapy can kill cancer cells, it doesn't finish off cancer stem cells—the very reason cancer can recur and spread throughout the body. The OPCs from this French grape seed extract eliminated cancer stem cells.

Other research has examined the effect of grape seed extract on breast cancer cells when used alone or with a conventional treatment. The results showed that the two interventions worked well together, but that grape seed extract alone was a strong inhibitor of breast cancer cells.

Researchers have also found that grape seed extract killed colon cancer cells outright. Other grape seed studies have shown that it stops prostate cancer cells through direct stimulation of tumor suppressing cells, and bladder cancer by increasing oxidative stresses only to cancer cells, halting their growth, while leaving healthy cells alone.

Lifesaving Power

I think we're going to see even more amazing results in the future when it comes to grape seed extract. This ingredient simply does it all! I urge everyone to take a French grape seed extract that is tannin-free and standardized to contain only small OPCs for the biggest benefits.

DOSAGE RECOMMENDATIONS

When it comes to grape seed extract, I recommend a French variety called VX1 above all others. Dosages for grape seed extract vary greatly, so it's best to check with your healthcare provider for specific recommendations. 150 mg daily is a beneficial amount to take for preventative measures, but some people take up to 400–1,200 mg per day to target acute conditions. For example, for high blood pressure I recommend 300 mg daily, and for cancer prevention I recommend 150–400 mg daily. For individuals hoping to slow tumor growth and the spread of cancer, I recommend 600–1,200 mg daily.

Green Tea—A Treasure Chest of Benefits

If you enjoy an occasional cup of tea, or even a few cups every day, you're not alone. Tea—second only to water—is the world's most commonly consumed beverage, and has been enjoyed as a drink and a natural medicine for about 5,000 years. First discovered in China, the plant was introduced to Japan, and by the 1200s, a Zen priest published "Tea and Health Promotion," outlining its cultivation and amazing benefits. It is clinically effective for heart, brain, cancer, and more.

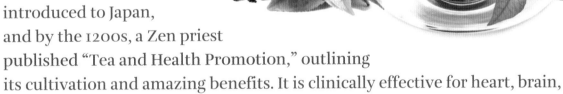

• •

All tea—black, green, oolong, white—is from the same plant, *Camellia sinensis,* and can share some of the same properties. But green tea—the leaves are steamed after harvest and very minimally processed—has amazing strength to prevent disease and keep us healthy.

Green tea is a rich source of natural compounds that protect you and help your mind and body function better. Among them are theanine (an amino acid known for its calming and focusing properties),

caffeine (at least in its drinkable form, and in some extracts), and catechins—chief among them, epic gallatin-3-gallate—better known as *EGCG.*

Catechins and other green tea compounds work on multiple fronts in the fight against cancer: they are strong anti-inflammatories and antioxidants that stop the DNA-damaging effects of oxidation and inflammation, prevent formation of cancer cells, and improve chemotherapy treatment.

Cancer Research

In a one year, double-blind, placebo-controlled study, 60 men at high risk of developing prostate cancer were provided with a green tea catechin (GTC) supplement or a placebo. The GTC supplement included a full spectrum of catechins and provided a naturally high level (over 50 percent) of EGCG.

By the end of the study, only one tumor (out of 30 participants) developed in the GTC group, while nine tumors developed in the placebo group. That puts the difference between green tea and placebo at three percent versus 30 percent, respectively. Those in the green tea group also reported higher quality of life scores and those with benign prostatic hyperplasia—BPH—better known as "enlarged prostate," noted fewer urinary symptoms, too.

A follow-up study two years later showed that green tea catechins *still* had a preventive effect; diagnoses of prostate cancer was reduced from 53 percent to 11 percent in the treatment group—a difference of almost 80 percent.

Other research with green tea consumption in Japan showed that the more cups of green tea per day that men drank, the less their risk of advanced prostate cancer. For those topping off at five or more cups per day, the risk was cut in half compared with less than one cup per day, so it shows that the amount really makes a difference.

If you love green tea, that's great news. However, if it's not for you, then definitely consider a high-quality extract standardized for a significant amount of EGCG. The compounds from green tea appear to stop tumor formation or growth by inhibiting cell-damaging inflammation and oxidation that would otherwise set up a spiral of poor cell replication. Simply affecting even *one* of these cancer-causing risks makes the odds much better for men.

Additionally, research shows that green tea may become an adjunct therapy along with conventional chemotherapy drugs, enhancing their effectiveness and reducing the drugs damage to liver cells.

For fighting other cancers, green tea shows a great deal of promise. It has been investigated for its effects on cervical cancer—with theanine, normally associated with the calming properties of green tea—being the principal active compound. Research has also found that green tea polyphenols and EGCG activate signals that lead to apoptosis—cancer cell death—of breast cancer cells and stops their proliferation.

Heart Disease and More

A Japanese study found that the more green tea individuals consumed, the less their odds of cardiovascular diseases, including stroke and coronary heart disease. While the effect was more pronounced in women than in men, it makes a strong case for incorporating green tea—or a strong extract—into your daily regimen. Other research and reviews have found that green tea appears to have an effect on reducing blood pressure in overweight or obese individuals.

Aside from these crucial abilities, green tea components also regulate blood sugar and help our metabolism burn calories properly and efficiently.

Healthy Weight Maintenance

In fact, while EGCG is often known as a cancer-preventing compound, it also activates pathways in the body that suppress the creation of fat cells, and stimulate the body's own abilities to break down fats. Additionally, a clinical study found that a high-dose green tea extract (with a high level of EGCG) helped women reduce waistlines and lower their BMI in 12 weeks because the EGCG affected hormone peptides that are related to weight gain.

Those in the high-dose green tea group showed reduced levels of ghrelin, known as the "hunger hormone" that helps send a signal that we need to eat—even when we don't really need to. The green tea group also had increased levels of adiponectin, a protein that moderates blood sugar levels and fat metabolism. In people who are overweight or obese, adiponectin levels are lower, potentially leading to problems with insulin resistance and a struggle to lose unwanted pounds. So it seems that green tea makes it easier for the body's own natural metabolism to work more effectively.

Another clinical study found that the best results from green tea on weight loss occurred when—not surprisingly—the treatment was combined with resistance training. However, both green tea groups —one exercising, the other not—still saw weight loss and a reduction in waist circumference and BMI. The addition of resistance training helped increase lean body mass (which tends to drive out fat accumulation), lower triglyceride levels, and build better muscle strength.

Alzheimer's Disease and Dementia

Green tea has also been studied for its ability to preserve the function of the brain. One of the biggest challenges to avoiding Alzheimer's disease (AD), dementia, or other forms of cognitive decline has been to keep inflammation and oxidation at bay in the delicate structure of the brain. As damage occurs in the brain, accumulated clusters of a protein called beta-amyloid— along with clumps of dying nerve and brain cells—disrupt the messages between neurons. Once the condition starts, it is difficult to slow or stop.

Studies with green tea extracts point in a positive direction. In a clinical study of individuals with severe AD, participants were provided with green tea extracts for two months. By the end of that period, researchers found that green tea helped the body produce protective antioxidants, including glutathione dismutase, considered the body's own "master antioxidant" and often considered a fountain of youth in its own right. It also significantly reduced the markers of stress that can begin or worsen the process of cognitive decline. Plus, green tea polyphenols also inhibit acetylcholinesterase, an enzyme that breaks down acetylcholine, a crucial, naturally occurring neurotransmitter.

I would encourage anyone to add green tea to their regimen. If the taste isn't for you, then consider a green tea supplement standardized for strong EGCG content.

DOSAGE RECOMMENDATIONS

I think that a daily maintenance level of 300 mg of a standardized green tea extract is appropriate. Studies have used short-term, high dosage levels of over 800 mg for weight loss and up to two grams per day for Alzheimer's research. Again, those were for brief periods, and not as a daily dose. It is truly a marvel of natural medicine for your body and mind.

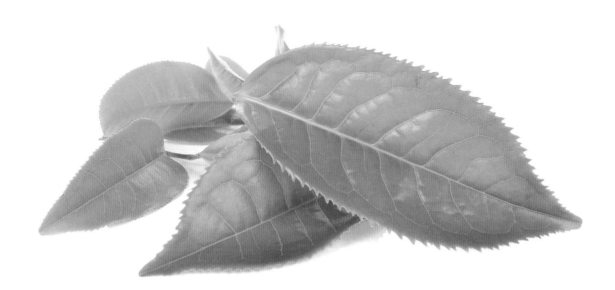

Hawthorn and the Heart

You may not know it, but Hawthorn is quite romantic. Hawthorn (*Crataegus* spp.) is a cousin to roses and shares in the symbolism of love and matrimony. In ancient Greece, you could find blossoming hawthorn sprigs entwined in wedding bouquets and worn as wedding crowns. In addition to its ornamental qualities, the medicinal usage of hawthorn was also documented in the first century. Hawthorn is one of the oldest and best-known herbal remedies for healing heart conditions—both physical and emotional. It is even rumored to mend a broken heart.

• •

In the early 19th century, American physicians treated respiratory and circulatory conditions with medicinal extracts made from the berries of this plant. With cardiovascular disease the primary cause of death in the United States, there is a great need for a heart-healthy herbal medicine like hawthorn.

Many Useful Medicines

Virtually every part of this sacred shrub is used to make medicinal preparations, including the berries, seeds, leaves, and flowers. Hawthorn naturally contains a variety of beneficial compounds including antioxidant flavonoids, oligomeric procyanidins (OPCs), and triterpenes. Hawthorn is commonly referred to as a heart "tonic," which is a substance that helps to restore vitality and functionality to the body, or a specific system in the body.

The name *Crataegus* is derived from the Greek word *kratos* meaning strength, and how fitting that this plant has been scientifically-studied for its ability to help the heart function more optimally during times of stress or disease. Integrative physicians have used hawthorn to help treat congestive heart failure (CHF), high blood pressure, palpitations, angina, heart rhythm issues, hardening of the arteries, and unbalanced cholesterol ratios.

Heart Research

A meta-analysis (reviewing data from multiple studies) of eight studies on hawthorn and patients with congestive heart failure provided substantial scientific evidence in favor of hawthorn. The authors noted that hawthorn significantly improved the heart's maximal workload (the heart's ability to function during exercise and other types of stress), enhanced the patients' ability to exercise, and positively influenced their quality of life, as measured by reductions in breathing difficulties and fatigue.

In a 2006 clinical study involving patients with type 2 diabetes and high blood pressure (hypertension), the participants receiving hawthorn extract at a dosage of 1,200 mg per day had very favorable results. The hawthorn group had significant reductions in their diastolic blood pressure versus placebo. Another encouraging discovery was that there were no interactions between hawthorn and the patients' diabetic prescription drugs. A separate study affirmed hawthorn's ability to lower diastolic blood pressure and also found a side benefit of anxiety reduction. Other studies have also shown that hawthorn can reduce both diastolic and systolic blood pressure.

Some of the key flavonoids in hawthorn include vitexin and hyperoside, so try and find a hawthorn extract that is standardized to these compounds.

DOSAGE RECOMMENDATIONS

The clinical research on hawthorn ranges from 300–1,800 mg per day. A good preventive dose would be 500 mg per day, while those looking for more serious support can try 1,000 mg once or twice daily.

Hemp Oil: The Emerging Science of Cannabinoids

For years, researchers and patients have experienced amazing effects from hemp compounds for everything from reducing seizures to stopping tumors. Until recently, the regulatory environment for anything from the *Cannabis sativa* plant has been unfriendly, and many people who would have benefited from the science and real-world results could not. Now they can.

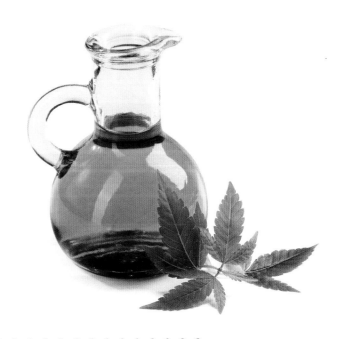

● ●

Hemp Oil is Not Marijuana

Before I go any further, I want to make it clear that what I am discussing is *not* marijuana. What hemp oil and marijuana have in common is that they originate from *Cannabis sativa*. But the plants themselves are different. Hemp oil is from industrial hemp plants selected to be high in non-psychoactive cannabinoids, while medical and recreational marijuana is from plants selected for THC

(delta-9-tetrahydrocannabinol) content, the compound that causes a "high." By law, hemp oil must contain less than 0.3 percent THC.

The *Cannabis sativa* stalks are extremely low in THC, but provide a full range of other compounds called cannabinoids, (including the popular cannabidiol (CBD), cannabinol, and cannabichromene) that affect the brain and body in very positive ways without impairing the focus of the person consuming it.

These compounds are also known as *phytocannabinoids* to distinguish them from naturally-occurring cannabinoids made in the body called *endocannabinoids*. These include anandamide (AEA) and 2-arachidonoylglycerol (2-AG), which affect emotions, the nervous and digestive systems, sensations of pain, and other aspects of health. These internally-created cannabinoids activate our receptors, and help us stay in a balanced, healthy state. In fact, anandamide is named for the Sanskrit word Ananda, which means bliss. That alone gives you a pretty good indication of how important the endocannabinoid system is to our well-being. It is essentially an adaptogenic system, affecting the body and mind in multiple ways.

Chronic disease, inflammation, stress, low omega-3 status, unbalanced diet, or a combination of these factors can deplete our endocannabinoids. Boosting our cannabinoid activity with phytocannabinoids can make an incredible difference. They can prevent the breakdown of our own natural cannabinoids, and research is finding that they can effectively treat a host of problems, from pain to cancer to epilepsy.

Cannabinoid Receptors & the Endocannabinoid System: A New Science

The science of cannabinoid receptors in what is called the *endocannabinoid system* (ECS) has really only been developed in the past 25 years or so.

If you notice a similarity between the words "cannabis" and "cannabinoid receptors", it is definitely not accidental.

This health system was discovered by doctors investigating the physical changes in the body in reaction to THC. Since THC is a cannabinoid, they called this a system of cannabinoid receptors. However, the system has existed for as long as there have been human beings.

These receptors, frequently abbreviated as CB1 and CB2, are involved with perception of pain, neurological functioning, *and* other physical health concerns, too. The compounds from cannabis interact with these receptors, found on the surfaces of cells. I think of them as light switches.

Both CB1 and CB2 are expressed in the hippocampus, a part of the brain associated with memory and emotion. This is part of the limbic system. But each also has its own areas of expertise, too. Broadly speaking, CB1 is involved with neurological responses—seizure, fear, and memory—while CB2 is more aligned with the immune system, peripheral structures of the body, and digestion. In an extremely simplified way, you could think of the CB1 receptor as the "mind receptor" and CB2 as the "body receptor". However, in truth, both play multiple roles.

Unfortunately, dietary deficiencies—including a lack of omega-3s, genetics, environment, and stress can rob us of our own endocannabinoids. That's where hemp oil compounds can help.

I think that the growing interest and research surrounding hemp oil is an exciting development in natural medicine, and one that is long overdue. Hemp oil has the potential to answer many serious health needs, and I'll review a few of them here.

Fights Pain and Inflammation

For fighting pain, I've often recommended curcumin enhanced with turmeric essential oil for better absorption, blood retention, and effectiveness. But hemp oil cannabinoids appear to be natural pain fighters due to their ability to reduce inflammation, too. In fact, it is one of the major reasons that people become interested in hemp oil in the first place. Of course, the reasons *why* the compounds from hemp oil fight pain is still under investigation.

Since hemp oil cannabinoids help preserve our own natural endocannabinoids, British research may provide a partial answer. They found that the synovial tissue (the tissue between the joints) in patients with osteoarthritis and rheumatoid arthritis had elevated levels of endocannabinoids compared to those *without* those conditions. It's as though the body was flooding those particular regions with endocannabinoids in order to relieve the pain.

Further research showed that changes in the endocannabinoid levels might also have something to do with the way we perceive pain, including feelings of anxiety and depression that often accompany joint conditions and a sense of immobility.

Phytocannabinoids may help people dealing with neuropathic pain from chemotherapy, which doesn't always respond easily to conventional medications. A double-blind, placebo-controlled pilot trial showed that an oral spray decreased pain by an average of 2.6 (compared to 0.6 for the placebo) on an 11-point pain intensity scale.

Other clinical work with oral sprays for neuropathic pain (which include THC and CBD) have found similar positive results.

The muscle spasticity in multiple sclerosis can also be difficult to treat with conventional drugs. A combination of THC/CBD improved conditions for some patients in as little as one month.

Fights Tumors

Phytocannabinoids from hemp have been found to kill cancer cells and inhibit the spread of tumors *without* affecting healthy cells.

For instance, CBD has been found to fight glioblastoma, a difficult-to-treat form of brain tumor. Researchers found that this compound found in hemp oil initially inhibited the spread of cancer cells, and seemed to work best when combined with conventional drugs in this scientific study. As we learn more, it's likely that cannabinoids from hemp could be considered an adjunct therapy for a variety of cancers.

The anti-inflammatory abilities of hemp oil are key to stopping cancer, although the exact pathways and exactly how it does this are still being investigated. It has been shown to reduce 5-lipoxygenase (5-LOX) inflammation, in one cell study by 40 percent, but there is still a lot of ongoing research in this area.

Scientific research has found that CBD also stops leukemia cells, while other work has found that a full range of cannabinoids inhibited prostate cancer, highlighting the value of a complete entourage of compounds from hemp.

Cannabinoids Reduce Seizures

One of the health concerns that could be most dramatically affected by cannabinoids from hemp oil is epilepsy. Epilepsy is a disorder in the central nervous system that disrupts the neural activity in the brain. The resulting symptoms of the condition can be as mild as a few unfocused seconds that would appear as daydreaming, to muscle twitches, to completely losing consciousness. Cannabidiol (CBD) from hemp has been clinically tested for individuals with the condition, and although more work needs to be done, initial results are very promising.

In an early clinical study, patients stayed on their anti-seizure medication (although the authors mentioned that it was no longer controlling symptoms) and took either CBD in hemp oil or a placebo. While there were only eight individuals taking the hemp oil compound, half of them were almost symptom free during the course of the trial, and three others noted a partial reduction in symptoms. This two-phase study began with small daily doses for the first 30 days (3 mg/kg), and followed with a larger dose (200–300 mg daily). This was one of the opening salvos in what would become a long road of using compounds from cannabis to promote health, without impairing or affecting cognition.

A more recent Israeli study found that a CBD-enriched hemp oil (which also included a small amount of tetrahydrocannabinol or "THC" in a ratio of 20:1 CBD to THC) reduced the frequency of seizures in 89 percent of the children in the trial. Of those, some (18 percent) saw a large drop in seizure frequency—anywhere from 75 to 100 percent. Researchers also reported improved language and motor skills, behavior, and sleep. The children included in this multi-center study had a form of epilepsy that was resistant to standard medications, so seeing positive results from hemp oil is a wonderful development.

What's interesting about the addition of a small level of THC in this case is that early research found that cannabidiol alleviates the "jitters" brought about in people by THC. The fact that CBD is considered an anticonvulsant and affects the brain and nerves in a stabilizing way may be one of the reasons it may combat drug-resistant seizures. More research will, no doubt, reveal more about the mechanism of action here. I think that combining hemp oil with a ketogenic diet, which has also been shown to decrease symptoms, could make a remarkable difference for those with epilepsy.

Hemp Oil Cannabinoids for Whole Body Health

In addition to the benefits I've outlined so far, cannabinoids from hemp oil may help strengthen your bones and keep your skin healthy, too.

Normally, specialized cells called osteoblasts add fresh minerals to bone while osteoclasts remove older bone tissue by breaking down the minerals and reabsorbing them into the bloodstream. The two processes are crucial for health and intricately interlinked. But age, diet, genetics, and a number of factors can create the conditions for osteoporosis and other bone-degenerative diseases. Aside from making sure you have a full calcium, mineral, and nutrient supplement in your regimen, you may want to add hemp oil.

Laboratory research at the Hebrew University in Jerusalem has found that hemp oil compounds helped heal bone fractures by stimulating osteoblast activity and helping build the matrix that supports minerals building new bone tissue. Considering the complications of many prescription drugs for dealing with bone issues, hemp oil provides a much better option.

Your endocannabinoid system regulates your skin, too. It regulates much of lipids (fats) that determines the oiliness or dryness of your skin and whether or not you suffer from dermatitis, acne, or other disorders. A supplemental hemp oil may help balance out your skin's production of oils.

Select the Best Hemp Oil

Hemp oil compounds, including CBD, have a lot to offer. But you have to be careful which kind you choose. It's easy to think that only CBD is important, but hemp oil is complex, and the other non-THC phytocannabinoids are incredibly valuable. The best hemp oil provides a full entourage of compounds, because a complete spectrum works together more strongly than any one single compound can on its own.

Also, be aware of the growing conditions of hemp oil. European, non-GMO hemp from specially cultivated plants that are carefully tended are going to deliver the results you're looking for. I would also suggest adding supplemental omega-3s to your diet, especially if they are bound to phospholipids. Omega-3s are part of the scaffolding for the endocannabinoid system, and phospholipids enhance the absorption and actions of hemp oil compounds.

I believe the highest quality hemp oil is obtained using a CO_2 extraction process. I also recommend looking for a hemp oil supplement in capsules or softgels—it's much more convenient than using a liquid dropper, and you can ensure that you're getting a consistent dosage each day.

There is a bright future for hemp oil. Like curcumin, French grape seed extract, and boswellia, it is an amazingly powerful natural medicine for almost every health condition.

CURCUMIN: A PERFECT PARTNER TO HEMP OIL

Hemp oil phytocannabinoids are amazing compounds. So are curcuminoids from turmeric. Pairing them up makes a lot of sense. These two botanicals fight pain, cancer, depression, Alzheimer's, and virtually double the protective power you can supply to your mind and body.

Your best option is a curcumin combined with turmeric essential oil for enhanced absorption, blood retention, and the added benefit of turmerones—compounds that have strong anti-inflammatory power of their own.

DOSAGE RECOMMENDATIONS

Full-spectrum hemp oil 50 mg, one to four capsules daily. You can adjust the dose as needed.

Hintonia Latiflora:
The Diabetes Miracle

The CDC reports that about 86 million Americans have prediabetes (high blood sugar, but not quite full blown diabetes) and 90 percent of them don't even realize it. That's in addition to the almost 30 million Americans who have diabetes, and another 25 percent who are not aware of it. There is a way to stop this epidemic.

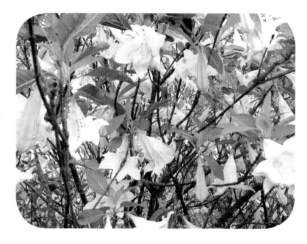

Hintonia latiflora grows in the deserts of Mexico and Central America, in a very harsh climate, which actually helps create the powerful defensive compounds in the plant that reduce high blood sugar.

• •

Type 1 diabetes is an autoimmune disease that generally occurs in childhood and early teen years. The immune system destroys the insulin-producing activity of the pancreas. However, about 90 percent of people with diabetes have type 2 diabetes. Type 2 diabetes is a metabolic disorder characterized by insulin resistance and eventually, reduced insulin production. It seems like the rise in type 2 diabetes has happened quickly, almost sweeping through the country like a virus. But that's not the case. All we have to do is look at our diets, and see that we've been building up to a diabetes epidemic for some time. In the space of about 70 years, we have dramatically increased our consumption of sugar, high fructose corn syrup, refined carbohydrates, (like white flour and white rice), and overly-processed foods. We have been setting ourselves up for a perfect storm of diabetes. And now it's arrived.

Hintonia—a Powerful Medicine

Along with the right diet and sensible exercise regimen, one of the best botanicals for anyone with elevated blood sugar or type 2 diabetes is *Hintonia latiflora.*

Hintonia latiflora is so well regarded that it has been clinically studied in Europe for over 60 years, and approved by doctors for use in people with type 2 diabetes. Almost from the beginning, early research showed that *Hintonia latiflora* could help people avoid the need to go on medication, or reduce medication in individuals unable to control their blood sugar by diet alone.

European Research

In a 2014 study published in the German journal *Naturheilpraxis mit Naturalmedizin* (*Naturopathic Practice with Natural Medicine*), the same dry concentrated bark extract of *Hintonia latiflora*—combined with additional nutrients—lowered A1C values (which show the average levels of blood sugar and are a way to gauge the control of diabetes), fasting glucose levels (blood sugar before a meal) and postprandial (after eating) blood sugar levels. Factoring all of the diabetic symptoms, the scores improved dramatically at the end of the study. Participants also saw improvements in blood pressure, lipids, and liver values.

Even a small change in A1C—and by small, I mean a one-point decrease—can mean huge improvements in health. By dropping it that tiny amount, you reduce the risk of cataracts by 19 percent, heart failure by 16 percent, and risk of amputation

or death from peripheral vascular disease by 43 percent.

In this study, after eight months, A1C levels improved by an average of almost 11 percent (nearly a full point)—a potentially life-saving difference. (Fasting glucose was lowered by an average of 23.3 percent, and postprandial (after meal) glucose by an average of 24.9 percent.)

Best of all, the herbal intervention was well tolerated—no one saw their blood sugar levels drop too low. And interestingly, individuals who were taking anti-diabetic prescription drugs stayed on their medication throughout the study. The *Hintonia* and nutrient combination was simply added on to their treatment. By the end of the study, 39 percent could reduce their medication dosages and some were able to stop their medication entirely.

In another clinical study, adult participants with type 2 diabetes were provided with the same extract of *Hintonia latiflora* also combined with trace nutrients (vitamins B1, B6, B12, folic acid, chromium, zinc, and vitamins C and E) for six months.

Once again, for fasting and postprandial blood glucose numbers and A1C levels, *Hintonia latiflora* significantly and clinically reduced these numbers. The study also showed that the botanical helped improve the cholesterol ratio and triglycerides.

How Does It Work?

The reason that Hintonia works is related to a compound in the bark, coutareagenin. This medicinal compound has many pathways by which it addresses blood sugar problems. According to research, one of its mechanisms is to inhibit alpha-glucosidase, an enzyme that releases sugar from carbohydrates.

Because *Hintonia* delays the release of sugar in the bloodstream, it keeps glucose balanced, rather than allowing it to spike as you see in cases of type 2 diabetes, or even in cases of hyper- and hypoglycemia. Another way it may normalize blood sugar is to help decrease insulin resistance and improve the function of the pancreas.

Blood Sugar and Brain

Aside from diabetes, the next major health crisis may be Alzheimer's disease. As it happens, the two are very likely linked. That's because glucose creates intensive inflammation in the brain. In fact, in one study, 25 percent of those with high blood sugar and diabetes developed Alzheimer's, which is a far greater number than the average non-diabetic population. Even just having high blood sugar in the "normal" range still led to an 18 percent increased risk of dementia.

It's understandable that there would be a connection. Elevated blood sugar causes inflammation in both the blood vessels and the soft tissue of the brain. There is already a well-documented connection between untreated elevated blood sugar and heart disease, kidney failure, and nerve and foot damage, so a possibility of it influencing Alzheimer's risk is not surprising. Hintonia can also normalize blood pressure levels that often rise due to the inflammatory effects of high blood sugar.

Even More Benefits

Aside from this, other *Hintonia* research shows that other compounds from the plant may help stop gastrointestinal damage and gastric ulcers. Considering the harshness of some drugs used for type 2 diabetes on the digestive system, this is yet another reason to consider adding *Hintonia latiflora* to a diabetes-fighting regimen.

Hintonia latiflora is a natural, tested, and effective botanical you can use with confidence with your existing regimen of diet, exercise, and supplementation. It has been shown to work well with conventional medications, and may even reduce your need for them. Hintonia has over six decades of study to back it up, and may be exactly the extra push you need to normalize your blood sugar levels for a vital, happy, and longer life.

DOSAGE RECOMMENDATIONS

I recommend you use the same botanical as the clinical studies, a *Hintonia latiflora* bark extract standardized for polyphenols. Start with 20 mg two times per day for controlling blood sugar levels, or increase to three times per day, if you are dealing with type 2 diabetes.

WHAT ARE "AIC LEVELS"?

You've heard of an A1C or HbA1C, but what is it, exactly? HbA1C is **hemoglobin** (a protein in red blood cells that carries oxygen throughout the body) that is joined to **glucose**. The **more sugar in your system, the higher your HbA1C levels** and the **higher your risk of diabetes**.

HbA1C levels show long-term trends in blood sugar (since HbA1C levels don't change quickly) versus blood glucose levels, which are only a "snapshot" of glucose levels at that moment.

According to the National Institute of Diabetes and Digestive and Kidney Diseases, most people need to at least keep their A1C levels below 5.7 percent to be in the normal range. If your range creeps up between 5.7 to 6.4 percent, you have prediabetes. At 6.5 and up, you have diabetes.

So lowering your A1C levels—even by 1 point—is an excellent step. **It can mean a 19 percent reduction in risk of cataracts**, a **16 percent reduction in risk of heart failure**, and a **43 percent less risk of amputation** or death from peripheral vascular disease.

The clinically studied *Hintonia latiflora* that I recommend has been shown to lower A1C levels by nearly a full point, and likely much more with a healthy diet, exercise, and ongoing use of Hintonia!

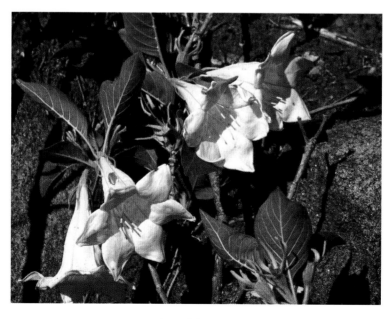

Holy Basil for Mind, Body and Spirit

Grown in India for more than 3,000 years, holy basil's use in the United States is a more recent occurrence. Also known as Tulsi, holy basil is historically said to benefit the mind, body, and spirit. Today, modern natural medicine is turning to holy basil as an effective tool to fight the damage that can happen in a world filled with stress.

• •

Not *That* Basil

Though closely related to sweet basil often used in cooking, holy basil (*Ocimum sanctum*) is a member of the mint, or Labiatae family and is not for culinary use. Holy basil has been the object of study as a natural medicine, with researchers trying to understand all that the herb can offer. Various parts of the plant including triterpenoic acids and eugenol have been studied for how they affect the immune system, reproductive system, central nervous system, cardiovascular system, gastric system, urinary system, and blood biochemistry. These studies have established a scientific basis for therapeutic uses of holy basil in such varied instances as being helpful after an initial cancer treatment to suppress secondary tumor formation and as a stabilizer for diabetes. The data that really stands out is the ability of holy basil to affect stress and aid in relaxation.

The Calming Effect

Holy basil contains natural compounds that alleviate stress and modulate adrenal reactions. It can be counted on to help the body adapt to stress and return more quickly to normal. When looking more closely at holy basil for this ability, it has been found to decrease stress hormone levels, in particular, corticosterone. Holy basil can be used to stop that "on alert" feeling without causing sedation—all while protecting the body from the damaging impact of oxidative stress.

In one study, scientists looked at noise induced oxidative stress. They weren't looking for the body's ability to simply get used to the noise or how it affected the subjects audibly, but rather how holy basil performed as an antioxidant against the elevated stress hormones induced by the noise. The phenolics and flavonoids in holy basil did the job by inhibiting the damaging effects of stress hormones in the brain.

As research on holy basil continues, we will find out more and more uses for this ancient wonder still held as sacred in India. For an extra avenue to dealing with stress, seek out a supplement that combines holy basil with lemon balm, which is an also excellent remedy for remaining relaxed, calm, and focused in our fast-paced world.

DOSAGE RECOMMENDATIONS

The best dosage is 500 mg of holy basil or as recommended by your health professional.

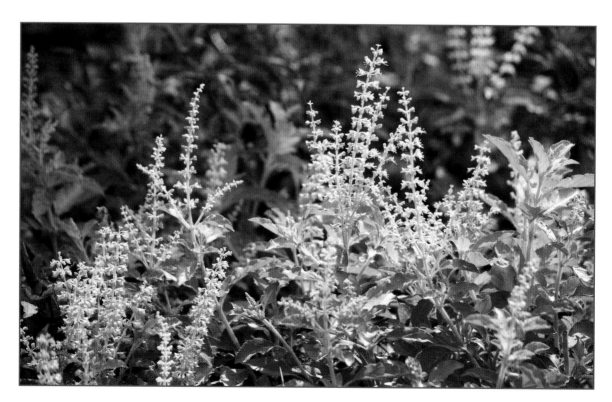

Iodine: The Thyroid Mineral

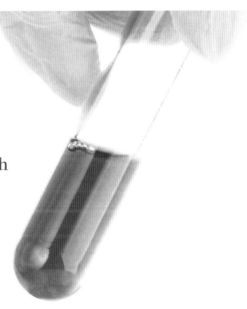

Iodine is one of nature's most amazing minerals. Your body needs it every day, yet most people don't get enough. That's because iodine is a trace element, meaning it's present in small amounts in the environment, and nearly impossible to obtain enough through the Standard American Diet. Some people believe they obtain the benefits of iodine through table salt, but the quality and absorbability of iodized table salt lends little benefit to improved health.

Deficiency from Toxic Exposure

People are also more iodine-deficient these days due to toxins in the environment. Chlorine, fluoride, and bromide—which lower iodine levels in the body by blocking iodine receptors—are increasingly consumed from foods and through environmental exposure. These minerals are detrimental to your thyroid and overall health. For example, fluoride blocks the ability of the thyroid gland to concentrate iodine, and bromide can cause depression and headaches.

In his book *Iodine: Why You Need It, Why You Can't Live Without It*, Dr. David Brownstein, M.D., states that about 90 percent of us lack sufficient iodine for optimal health, according to his tests on more than 5,000 patients. I'm convinced everyone can benefit from daily iodine supplementation. Iodine is known for supporting healthy thyroid function, as well as maintaining healthy breast, ovary, uterus, and prostate tissue. Researchers believe iodine can prevent cysts, nodules, and cancer, and that it has the ability to destroy bacteria and viruses.

Thyroid Health

Your thyroid gland is extremely important to your overall health and requires sufficient levels of iodine to function normally. Thyroid hormones regulate everything from metabolism to heart rate to brain function. When these hormones get out of balance; you may end up with hypothyroid or hyperthyroid symptoms, which can negatively impact countless aspects of your health and even cause autoimmune issues, including Hashimoto's and Grave's diseases.

One of the main functions of the thyroid is the production of the hormone thyroxine (T4), and the conversion of this hormone into triiodothyronine (T3) as needed for metabolism and weight management. These hormones are made from tyrosine (an amino acid) and iodine. Without sufficient iodine, the thyroid simply can't manufacture these very important hormones.

Cancer Prevention

Iodine's anti-cancer functions are one of its most important benefits. Scientific tests using estrogen-sensitive breast cancer cells exposed to iodine have shown that they are less likely to grow and spread. It is also beneficial for the prevention of thyroid, prostate, uterine, and ovarian cancer.

How Iodine Promotes Breast and Prostate Health

Iodine works so well for breast health because it makes breast cells less sensitive to estrogen, and as mentioned earlier, detoxifies toxic halogens—bromide, fluoride, and chlorine—from the body. It's important that you help your body flush out these harmful elements: one study found that breast cancer patients had double the bromide levels compared to non-cancer patients.

For the same reasons, iodine helps prevent the hormonal imbalances that leave some men more prone to prostate cancer. After all, women and men are equally subject to the estrogen-like chemicals in the environment. These chemicals are prevalent in modern packaging, home and office furnishings, and foods.

Iodine also improves fibrocystic breast disease. In clinical research, approximately 70 percent of patients experienced relief of pain and reduction in abnormal tissue with iodine supplementation. In patients with mastalgia (breast pain), at least 50 percent of the women had significant reductions in breast pain after taking 6 mg of iodine each day. In another study, 98 percent of women receiving iodine treatment were pain free by the study's end, and 72 percent had improvements in breast tissue.

Different Forms of Iodine for Different Reasons

Supplemental iodine is available in different forms, each of which affects specific tissues in the body. Potassium and sodium iodide are best absorbed by the thyroid. Breast tissue uses iodine most efficiently in the form of molecular iodine.

Because of this, you need a supplement that includes more than one form of the mineral. The best formula provides three forms of iodine—sodium iodide, potassium iodide, and molecular iodine—at levels that can actually make a noticeably positive difference.

How much should you take? Dr. Brownstein states, "As I started to use larger amounts of iodine (12.5–50 mg/day) to achieve whole body sufficiency, I began to see positive results in my patients. Goiters and nodules of the thyroid shrank, cysts on the ovaries became smaller and began to disappear, patients reported increased energy, and metabolism was increased as evidenced by my patients having new success in losing weight. Libido improved in both men and women. People suffering from brain fog reported a clearing of the fogginess. Patients reported having vivid dreams and sleeping better. Most importantly, those with chronic illnesses that were having a difficult time improving began to notice many of their symptoms resolving."

Iodine supplementation can make a big difference to your health. Boost your metabolism, protect your thyroid, and overcome cancer risk by adding it to your daily regimen.

DOSAGE RECOMMENDATIONS

The most common dosages are 6.25–12.5 mg, but doctors sometimes recommend higher or lower in certain health conditions. For maximum thyroid impact, iodine should be taken with L-tyrosine and selenium.

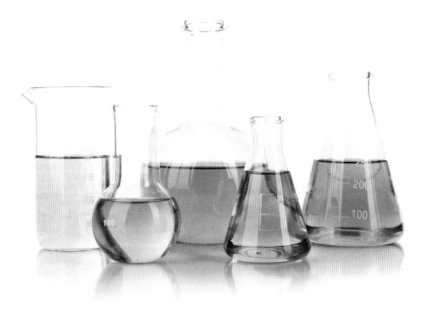

Melissa, or Sweet Melissa, for a Sweet Life

Melissa (*Melissa officinalis*), or lemon balm, is a lemon-scented herb that has been used medicinally for centuries. The oil is popular in aromatherapy for everything from sharpening the memory to erasing wrinkles, and herbalists often use it to treat cold and flu viruses because of its potent antiviral and antibacterial properties. While it's an effective remedy for a wide range of health concerns, Melissa is one of my favorite herbs for its ability to treat anxiety, stress, and insomnia.

• •

Melt Away the Effects of Stress

Melissa acts as an effective calming agent and a mild sedative, making it perfect for times when your nerves get the best of you. It is also an efficient sleep aid, proven to be effective for those who need help falling asleep and staying asleep.

Participants using lemon balm in an open-label clinical study noticed significant reductions in stress-related concerns. In just two weeks, volunteers between the ages of 18 and 70 who received a special extract twice daily saw their stress levels drop significantly. In fact, 95 percent of the participants responded to the treatment, with 70 percent achieving full recovery from anxiety and 85 percent experiencing less insomnia. Participants reported no adverse side effects to the lemon balm, unlike many prescription drugs.

Scientific studies have shown that lemon balm may bind to gamma-aminobutyric acid (GABA) receptors, helping the nervous system to calm down. GABA is a neurotransmitter that helps stop anxiety and sleeplessness. In a double-blind, placebo-controlled British study, healthy volunteers in the Melissa treatment group significantly improved their cognitive function and calmness ratings compared to placebo. What's more, the calmness lasted the remainder of the testing day.

Yet another study—completed in Australia—found that lemon balm extract improved mood and cognitive function in volunteers performing multiple tasks. The researchers pointed to rosmarinic acid in the lemon balm as the prime cause of the effects.

Chronic stress can weaken your immune system, leaving you vulnerable to a whole host of diseases. Melissa is a fantastic botanical for helping to improve sleep quality and reduce the negative effects that stress can have on your health.

DOSAGE RECOMMENDATIONS

The amount of Melissa you should take varies based on your unique needs, but common doses range from 300–500 mg, up to three times daily.

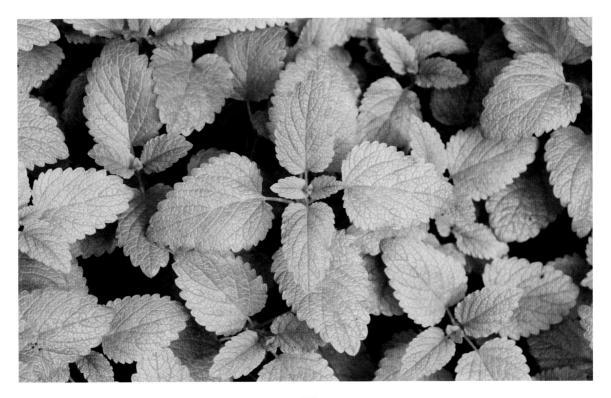

Mesoglycan: Reopen, Repair, Rebuild Blood Vessels

Mesoglycan is produced naturally by the body and rebuilds and restores our blood vessels. The three types of blood vessels in the body are arteries (carry blood away from the heart), veins (carry blood back to the heart), and capillaries (the smallest blood vessels in our body). An average adult contains over 60,000 miles of 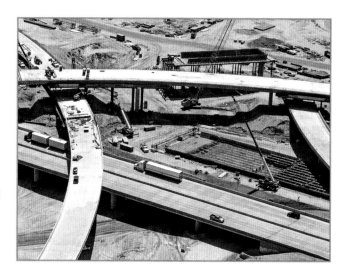 blood vessels in our circulatory system that are working around the clock to deliver nutrients and oxygen while also removing waste materials. Just like frequently traveled highways, sometimes potholes and road repairs need to take place.

• •

Mesoglycan and Heart Disease

With heart disease remaining as the number one cause of death in the United States, now more than ever we need to fortify our defenses against this widespread killer. We know that quitting smoking, diet, and exercise play a huge role, but what about correcting the damage that has already been done? This is an area of great concern, because this type of injury results over many years, or even decades, so the problem cannot be corrected overnight. Heart disease can be caused by a variety of factors including high blood pressure, oxidative stress, chronic inflammation, and diseases like diabetes. Regardless of the cause, I think mesoglycan is one of the best compounds for rebuilding and repairing our cardiovascular system.

Conventional medications used to treat cardiovascular conditions generally focus on a certain pathway in the body, but without treating the underlying cause of the disease. However, mesoglycan is able to restructure our blood vessels naturally to make them more flexible and resistant to disease.

Atherosclerosis

One of the early signs of heart disease is a condition called atherosclerosis, which means hardening of the arteries. As toxins and irritating substances wreak havoc on the inside of the blood vessels, the body sends repair substances like cholesterol and calcium to patch things up. So while cholesterol is used as a bandage, it often gets blamed as the cause of heart disease, which is simply not the case. Over time, this on-going repair process can make the blood vessels more stiff and rigid, causing them to lose their elasticity. They also become narrower, and more likely to trap a blood clot, leading to a heart attack, stroke, or deep vein thrombosis (DVT).

An Italian study looking at mesoglycan's effects on hardening of the arteries had very favorable results in just 18 months. When compared to the mesoglycan group, the control group had more than a seven-fold increase in the thickening of their arteries. The mesoglycan group received a mere 200 mg per day of this life-changing natural medicine. Such a drastic decrease can have a multitude of benefits in the body.

Did you know that artery thickening can also contribute to high blood pressure?

Imagine a hose that has water pumping through it. Now think about what happens to the water flow when the inner part of the hose starts to thicken, it becomes much more difficult for the water to pass through. This is exactly what happens to the interior of our blood vessels after extensive damage. More resistance in the blood vessels forces the heart to work harder, causing a lot more wear and tear. So you may want to consider mesoglycan as part of your high blood pressure prevention or treatment regimen as well.

Stroke Prevention

Several human studies have explored mesoglycan's benefits for people suffering from cerebrovascular disease (reductions in blood circulation to the brain), often called a stroke. Generally, patients suffering from cerebrovascular disease have to go on blood-thinners or other dangerous medications for the rest of their life. Mesoglycan offers a much safer alternative, while still providing life-changing benefits.

One human study found that mesoglycan was just as effective as the standard treatment. The patients in the mesoglycan group were given a total of 100 mg per day. Both the mesoglycan and treatment groups had similar outcomes for the amount of ischemic (restriction in blood flow) incidences and improvements in quality of life.

Another study involving patients with moderate to severe cerebrovascular disease also demonstrated positive results. The study lasted six months, but significant improvements were already seen after only three months. The patients receiving 100 mg of mesoglycan per day demonstrated improvements in their behavior and cognition. This is a very important finding because impaired blood flow to the brain can cause mood and memory changes.

Diabetic Retinopathy

Sugar is probably the most irritating substance to the inside of our blood vessels. So it makes sense that people with diabetes often have higher levels of heart disease, kidney disease, and retinopathy. Some of the tiniest blood vessels in the body are found in our eyes. When chronic inflammation from elevated blood sugar occurs within those tiny blood vessels, they can bulge and tear, which impairs the body's ability to nourish the retina. This results in a leading cause of blindness, diabetic retinopathy.

A 2012 study using 100 mg of mesoglycan per day for six months showed a significant improvement in the patient's retinopathy. The mesoglycan group had fewer incidents of blood vessel swelling (microaneurysm) and leaking (microhemorrhage). While no one in the placebo group experienced clinical improvement after six months, almost everyone in the mesoglycan group did.

This is great news for the millions of Americans who suffer from diabetes. Mesoglycan can help to not only preserve eyesight, but also assist with proper circulation throughout the entire body.

Additional Benefits of Mesoglycan

While mesoglycan's effects may be best known for correcting cardiovascular issues, everything in our body is nourished by blood vessels. Other conditions for which mesoglycan usage has been scientifically validated include deep vein thrombosis, chronic venous insufficiency, Raynaud's phenomenon, intermittent claudication, peripheral artery disease, varicose veins, hemorrhoids, leg edema (swelling), and many others.

Mesoglycan supplements are derived from an animal source because it is the most similar to the mesoglycan that is found in the human body.

DOSAGE RECOMMENDATIONS

The majority of studies used between 50–100 mg of oral mesoglycan per day, though some increase to 200 mg.

Myrtle: A Mighty Oil

No one can say exactly where the myrtle shrub comes from, although its medicinal properties are well known throughout the Mediterranean, Middle East, and North Africa. A very sturdy and hardy evergreen, myrtle is also very fragrant. Myrtle is used as a spice in food preparation, in liquors, and as a fragrance for perfumes. Through the centuries people have also turned to myrtle as medicine for a variety of ailments including diarrhea, ulcers, inflammation, skin diseases, hemorrhoids, cancer, and diabetes. Today, the oil from the leaves of the myrtle shrub have been studied and shown to provide powerful antibacterial activities to fight a variety of respiratory infections.

• •

A Long History of Health

Myrtle (*Myrtus communis cineole*), as myrtle oil, has been sold in Europe for over 75 years.

From ancient times until today, myrtle has remained a constant because of its expectorant, decongestant, astringent, anti-inflammatory, and antimicrobial properties. Myrtle has been well studied for the ability to stimulate the cilia in the respiratory system and sinus cavities, brushing the mucus out of those areas and clearing congestion. That ability is due to a powerful compound in the plant oil called 1,8 cineole. Working as an antiseptic and antibacterial agent, myrtle oil is an excellent choice for treating bronchial and sinus issues. One study, in particular, found that Myrtle essential oil was significantly superior at treating sinusitis symptoms compared to a placebo.

Go for the Power

A component that works well with myrtle oil is eucalyptus oil, which also contains 1,8 cineole and other strong anti-inflammatory compounds. For a very effective combination against respiratory ailments, seek a supplement that offers both eucalyptus and myrtle oils. An important point to remember is that myrtle and eucalyptus oil designed for internal use is not the same as the oils used in aromatherapy. Oils for internal use are up to 100 times more concentrated than dry herbal extracts and verified for the correct plant, species, botanical markers, and demonstrated human safety. Myrtle oil for internal use is potent medicine. Make sure that any plant oils you use for clearing sinuses and infections are meant to be taken internally and have been examined and certified to be the correct plant species, containing the beneficial key compounds. Since there are over 2,800 varieties of myrtle, you want to know that you are getting the best compounds from the best species that have been tested for purity. To remain clear and breathing deeply, myrtle is the clear answer.

DOSAGE RECOMMENDATIONS

Take 25–50 mg of myrtle leaf oil, up to six times daily. Look for myrtle leaf oil in a softgel that contains 20–60 percent alpha-pinene, 15–35 percent 1,8 cineole, along with the 1,8 cineole eucalyptus oil. Essential oils are generally very low dose due to their high concentration of compounds. If it is blended with another oil, make sure it is in a base of extra virgin olive oil for best health benefits.

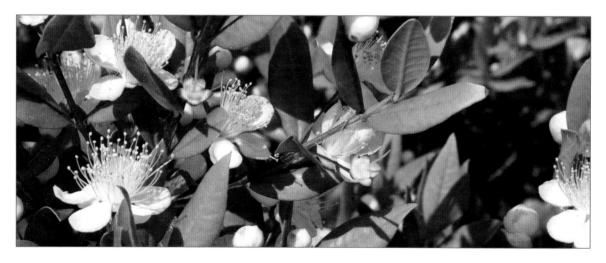

Olive: The Tree of Life

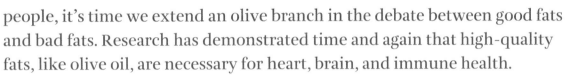

Olive trees have been cultivated in the Mediterranean for over 7,000 years. Their versatility—food, lumber, decoration, religion, medicine—has made olive trees one of the most renowned and revered plants in the world.

Around 90 percent of the world's olives are used to produce olive oil. While diets rich in fats and oils are controversial to some people, it's time we extend an olive branch in the debate between good fats and bad fats. Research has demonstrated time and again that high-quality fats, like olive oil, are necessary for heart, brain, and immune health.

• •

Health Benefits

Olives may be best known for their role in protecting the cardiovascular system. Clinical studies have found that olive oil and its extracts can balance cholesterol, regulate genes associated with athero-sclerosis and intimal thickening, increase blood vessel function, and improve blood pressure.

Olive oil may garnish much of the fame and glory, but there are many other health-promoting compounds that the olive tree provides. Extracts of olive fruit, leaf, and fruit oil concentrate often contain other compounds that are not always found in olive oil. While olives contain hundreds of natural compounds, oleuropein is certainly one of the most powerful and is generally more concentrated in the leaves. Hundreds of scientific studies have evaluated oleuro-pein for health conditions including cancer, oxidative stress and inflammation, diabe-tes, aging, bacterial illnesses, Alzheimer's disease, and many others.

An olive leaf extract standardized to 16–24 percent oleuropein has been clinically studied for its effects on blood pressure. In a study involving patients with stage 1 hypertension, participants were given either olive leaf extract or the prescription antihypertensive Captopril. After eight weeks, both groups experienced significant reductions in their systolic and diastolic blood pressure. Additionally, the olive extract group experienced a significant reduction in their triglycerides, while the Captopril group did not.

Other compounds in olive leaf and fruit extracts include oleanolic acid, tyrosol/hydroxytyrosol, tocopherols, triterpenic compounds, oleic acid (omega-9 fatty acid), and beta-sitosterol.

Oil vs Supplement

When using olives for culinary purposes, like cooking, I think olive oil can be an excellent choice. However, olive oil can be very inconsistent when it comes to purity and quality. Plus, olive extracts contain significantly fewer calories for those who are on a calorie-restricted diet or people with diabetes. For example, olive oil is about 238 calories for two tablespoons and a good olive extract can provide excellent benefits with about five calories per 160 mg dose.

When you are looking for consistent levels of key compounds like oleuropein and polyphenols, I think an olive extract is a better choice.

DOSAGE RECOMMENDATIONS

Concentrated olive extract, 160 mg once or twice daily. If using olive oil, take 2 to 4 Tbsp. once or twice daily.

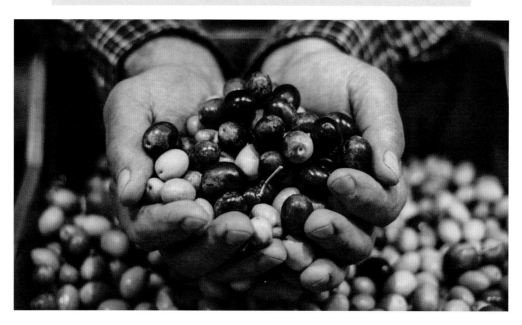

Omega-3 Fatty Acids from Salmon

When your doctor tells you that you need to eat more fish or take a fish oil product, what they're really telling you is that you need more omega-3s. Omega-3s are healthy, polyunsaturated fats, also referred to as essential fatty acids or EFAs. They're called "essential" because you need to get them from dietary sources—your body can't make them on its own. Fish oil is the transporter of omega-3s, but they are not the same thing.

Omega-3s are highly valued for their anti-inflammatory properties and abilities to support heart, brain, and skin health. More specifically, they can help to alleviate depression, boost cognitive ability, keep emotions on an even keel, build strong and flexible blood vessels and arteries, and reduce inflammation throughout the body.

Supplementation of omega-3s can be complicated. With fish oil, there are a lot of variables, not the least of which is the quality of the oil itself, level of rancidity, and how well it's actually absorbed and used by the body. Krill oil, another common source of omega-3s, is prone to rancidity and not sustainable. I recommend a strong phospholipid-bound omega-3 fatty acid supplement from salmon. It is not a fish oil, but a bioidentical extract that provides the added benefits of phospholipids and peptides. It contains DHA, the preferred fatty acid for cognitive development, as well as EPA. Both these fatty acids play a multitude of important roles in the body.

Phospholipids and Peptides

Phospholipids are what help your body absorb and use omega-3s. They're also useful on their own. They protect the mitochondria—the "engine" of your cells—from oxidative damage, and can help your hearing and vision stay healthy and sharp. Phospholipids also help build the myelin sheath that surrounds your nerve cells, keeping those signals firing properly, and helps keep your brain healthy and your mood positive.

Peptides are short, beneficial chains of amino acids that protect delicate blood vessels in the brain by fighting oxidative damage. They're not found in fish oil or krill oil. One scientific study found these peptides to significantly reduce anxiety over the course of 14 days.

The combination of phospholipids and peptides in the salmon extract I recommend enables omega-3s to deliver dramatic results to various parts of your body.

Boosts Brain Power

DHA and phospholipids make up a great deal of our brain. In fact, the brain itself is about 60 percent fat, and 15 to 20 percent of the fat in the brain is DHA. The brain needs phospholipids and DHA to develop properly and age well. In fact, phospholipids have been shown to combat depression and other neurological disorders.

In an in-vitro study in the *Journal of Neurochemistry,* researchers pre-treated neuronal cells with DHA from a phospholipid-bound omega-3 source. Forty eight hours later, they exposed the cells to soluble oligomers of amyloid-beta peptide, which are known to cause the brain cell damage associated with Alzheimer's disease. The study had an intriguing result: the DHA

pretreatment greatly increased cell survival and reduced damage. Researchers concluded the study to be of major interest in the prevention of Alzheimer's and other neurodegenerative diseases.

Supports Heart Health

Omega-3s slow the formation of plaque, prevent inflammation, and keep arteries flexible for better blood flow and therefore, lower blood pressure. They are effective at preventing abnormal blood clots that can trigger heart attacks and strokes, and they reduce inflammation that can lead to clogged arteries.

Clinical trials prove that omega-3s can also help to keep cholesterol in balance by boosting HDL levels and lowering LDL and triglyceride levels. In one study, triglycerides were reduced in people who were given more omega-3s than what is typically found in a serving of cold water fatty fish.

In another study, 40 healthy volunteers took two tablets of phospholipid-bound omega-3 fatty acid salmon extract per day without any modifications to diet or exercise habits. After 60 days, the participants saw their triglyceride levels drop by 16 percent, and their HDL levels—the "good cholesterol"—increase by 13 percent. There were also very significant improvements in C-reactive protein (CRP) a measure of ongoing inflammation.

I don't think that there is any doubt that omega-3s should be a foundational supplement in virtually everyone's daily health plan, but remember that the delivery system is key for optimal benefits.

DOSAGE RECOMMENDATIONS

Remember to look for an omega-3 salmon extract that contains both phospholipids and peptides. Because these formulas are more effective than fish and krill oil, you should only need approximately 300 mg to 600 mg daily, but it is perfectly safe to increase your dosage for maximum benefits.

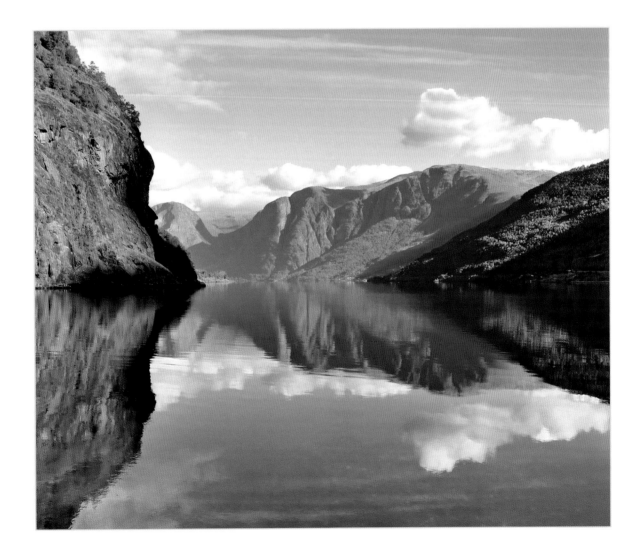

Oregano:
Much More Than a Seasoning

Most people enjoy oregano as a seasoning and ingredient. There are various types of oregano that have been studied worldwide, but whatever the species, they all share some basic compounds that can stop bacteria, boost your immune system's response, act as a natural food preservative, and possibly even stop the development of cancer cells.

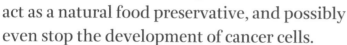

Scientific research found that oil of oregano—*Origanum vulgare*—the species many of us are familiar with and probably have in our kitchens—was able to inhibit the bacteria responsible for typhoid. The researchers found that by combining oregano with a common medication for typhoid, ciprofloxacin, it enhanced the ability of the medication and may potentially reduce side effects, too. This is critically important—not only for those at risk of that specific disease (which if left untreated, can have a mortality rate of up to 30 percent), but because like so many antibiotics, ciprofloxacin is succumbing to the same antibiotic resistance and becoming less useful.

A Replacement for Antibiotics?

Antimicrobial action is one of the key reasons that research of oregano oil is considered so urgent. Some of this work is simply investigating which species have the highest concentrations of specific compounds, including carvacrol and thymol. The results have shown that oregano oil fights some of the most dangerous infectious bacteria, including *Staphylococcus aureus* (staph infections) and *Escherichia coli* (potentially deadly food poisoning), and many others.

Worldwide Research

For example, Italian research showed that essential oil from oregano dramatically inhibited bacterial strains that are dangerous for individuals with cystic fibrosis, a condition with a serious burden on the lungs and immune system and carries a great susceptibility to infections.

Essential oil from Moroccan oregano (*Origanum compactum*) has also been the focus of intensive research because it also provides high levels of carvacrol and thymol and shows strong antibacterial actions against *Staphylococcus aureus* and *Escherichia coli.* Considering the damage that just these two bacteria cause each year—ranging from skin irritation and milder symptoms to emergency room treatment—this is good news, and more evidence of the herb's amazing value to natural medicine.

And, at Georgetown University, researchers concluded that oregano oil used alone or in combination with mono-laurin (which can be derived from coconut oil) is highly effective against bacteria, including *E. coli* and *H. pylori* (responsible for chronic gastritis and ulcers). The authors concluded that due to the safety record of these natural interventions, oregano oil might help prevent and treat severe bacterial infections, especially those that are difficult to treat or are resistant to antibiotics. In fact, the carvacrol in oregano oil was just as effective as antibiotics. Considering how overused antibiotics have become (and as a result, virtually useless in some applications), this proves that much of what we really need can be found in nature.

Along with strong bacterial inhibition, *Origanum compactum* appears to inhibit breast cancer cells. While further study is necessary, it shows the exciting potential of this widely-used medicinal plant.

A Pharmacy Unto Itself

I think the concentrated essential oil of oregano is practically a pharmacy unto itself. Whether you simply want to bolster your immune system and cellular defenses, or you're facing cold and flu season and serious risk of bacterial infections, this outstanding botanical ingredient is a must.

DOSAGE RECOMMENDATIONS

Taking 150 mg once daily can keep your immune system on track. If you're already dealing with an illness, consider taking 150 mg three or four times daily for no more than one week.

Pomegranate: A Treasure from the Garden of Eden

If you want to talk about a fruit that has received a lot of attention in the past few years, that's pomegranate. Said to have originated in agriculture as early as 3500 B.C., it is the fruit spoken of in many ancient texts, including the Bible. In fact, many scholars say the fruit in the Garden of Eden was, in fact, a pomegranate. The ancient Greeks believed the seasons were divided because the kidnapped daughter of the earth goddess Demeter ate six seeds of the pomegranate, and was forced to live in the underworld six months of the year. Her mother's grief resulted in winter. Shakespeare used the pomegranate as a symbolism for love in *Romeo and Juliet.* Today we know that the pomegranate offers much more than metaphors and myths. Officially considered a berry, this fruit, revered for thousands of years, has a wealth of health to provide us today.

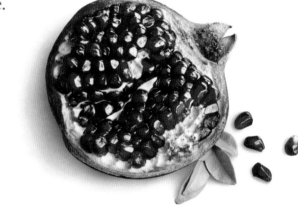

• •

A More Recent Hit

If you don't remember growing up eating pomegranates like you did bananas, that's because in the year 2000, only four percent of Americans had ever tasted a pomegranate! It wasn't until 2007 that an ad campaign began to introduce the pomegranate to the public as a fruit full of promise, rather than an unknown entity on the fruit shelf. This set off interest for more farmers to grow pomegranates, which started a domino effect of supply and demand.

Pomegranates (*Punica granatum*) come from a bushy tree that can grow as high as 25 feet, but is more typically 12–16 feet. The blossoms come in spring with appealing orange-red flowers. At harvest, the bell-shaped fruit with the red leathery skin offers a host of eating and drinking options. Slice one open and you'll see smaller fleshy seeds called "arils" that provide the popular pomegranate juice and are a good source of dietary fiber. Seed numbers vary in the fruit ranging from 200 to 1400. The arils are also enjoyable on their own or in smoothies, in baking, cooking, and even as part of other juices or wines. To eat a pomegranate, score it with a knife and break it open. An easier way to separate the seeds is to submerge it in a bowl of water, causing the seeds to sink and the pulp to float. Another tip is to freeze your whole pomegranate before cutting it.

The fruit has become highly popular for juice, and not just for the flavor, but also because of research showing its ability to provide strong antioxidant protection for the cardiovascular system, reduce inflammation, protect joint cartilage, and more.

Getting the Most Powerful Option

While pomegranate juice has many health benefits, it's also high in calories and sugar. That makes it difficult to consume enough juice to have a therapeutic effect. Plus, by only drinking the juice, you're missing out on some of the most important compounds in the plant. For optimum benefits, zero in on the power of the pomegranate fruit and seed oil, which has the only known botanical source of omega-5 fatty acid, also

known as punicic acid. Utilizing this combination of a fruit and seed oil extract, rich in omega-5 fatty acids has been shown to:

- Stop tumors in breast, colon, and prostate cells
- Cause breast cancer cells to self-destruct
- Fight inflammation and oxidation
- Promote healthy aging
- Stop damage to joints and cartilage
- Boost the immune system
- Preserve and strengthen heart function

Pomegranate and Breast Cancer

In looking closer at just one of the topics greatly affected by pomegranate seed oil, it has been shown that the omega-5 in the oil can inhibit both estrogen-sensitive and estrogen insensitive breast cancer cells. In fact, in a cellular study, the omega-5 from the pomegranate seed oil inhibited proliferation of two types of cancer cells by 92 and 96 percent, respectively. In that same study, omega-5 fatty acid (punicic acid) also supported apoptosis (cancer cell death) in two types of breast cancer cells, by 86 and 91 percent. As an aromatase inhibitor (aromatase is an enzyme that affects the body's steroid metabolism), pomegranate seed oil extract was found to inhibit aromatase activity by 60 to 80 percent. This same study also found that pomegranate seed oil showed a 90 percent inhibition of MCF-7 breast cancer cells. The researchers stated that pomegranate has excellent chemopreventive potential, either on its own or as an addition to conventional therapy, which can mean less dependence on dangerous drugs. Choose a pomegranate supplement with organic pomegranate seed oil using a supercritical CO_2 extraction standardized to contain punicic acid, the unique, very important Omega-5 fatty acid, and standardized pomegranate fruit extract.

The research is clear; the mighty pomegranate is here to stay with answers for many of today's health concerns.

DOSAGE RECOMMENDATIONS

If you are using a powder extract, the dosage is 200–400 mg each day. However, I like the combination of pomegranate seed oil with the fruit extract for a wider spectrum of effective compounds. A good dose is 500–1,000 mg of pomegranate seed oil.

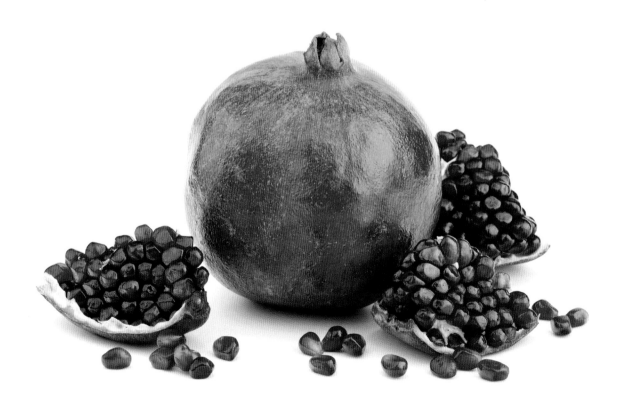

Probiotics:
Digestive Health and More

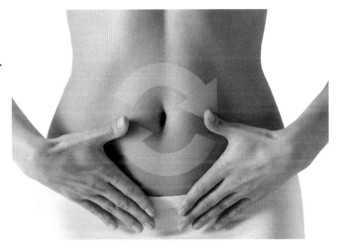

To say that your digestion is connected to all other facets of your health is no exaggeration. Without the ability to properly assimilate nutrients, you can't fight disease, stop oxidative damage to your cells, or fuel your body and mind. So keeping the digestive system running smoothly and stopping the dysfunction that leads to conditions such as irritable bowel syndrome (IBS), Crohn's disease, colitis, and other inflammatory bowel diseases (IBD) is crucial. One of the best ways to do that is with probiotics—healthy bacteria that naturally reside in your digestive system and are extremely beneficial to your health.

- -

Lactobacillus plantarum for Gas, Bloating, and C. Diff

One of the most extensively tested probiotics, *Lactobacillus plantarum*, has wide-ranging benefits. In clinical studies, it has been found to reduce gas, abdominal pain, bloating, and other symptoms of IBS.

Other research has explored the ability of this powerful probiotic to reduce the incidence of a condition known as *Clostridium difficile (C-Diff)*-associated disease. It occurs most often in hospitalized patients who have been treated with antibiotics. It is notoriously difficult to treat.

The reason this probiotic is so effective is because it is especially equipped to survive the trip through the acid environment of the stomach and adhere to the mucosa—the inner walls of the intestine—where it can colonize and multiply.

Lactobacillus rhamnosus for IBD, Leaky Gut, and Crohn's Disease

Another probiotic bacteria, *Lactobacillus rhamnosus*, is well known for its ability to stop the conditions that lead to inflammatory bowel disease (IBD). A Spanish review examined the ways that probiotics address the symptoms of IBD, and named it as one of the probiotics that reduce inflammatory conditions in the digestive tract. This same review also mentioned that because *L. rhamnosus* appears to reduce inflammation, it can strengthen the barrier in the intestines to prevent leaky gut (the leaching of large food particles from the digestive tract into the bloodstream).

Right now, conventional wisdom says that there is no cure for Crohn's disease or ulcerative colitis. But with probiotics, an effective, long-term answer is closer than you think. Even if you don't have IBD, this probiotic can stop the inflammation in your digestive tract that can cause gas, bloating, and loose stools. Also, *L. rhamnosus* may help prevent more serious conditions from developing down the road.

Bifidobacterium bifidum for IBS

In clinical trials, *Bifidobacterium bifidum* has been found to significantly reduce IBS symptoms—including pain and discomfort, the frequency of bowel movements, urgency, and bloating—while improving the overall quality of life. It is thought to be especially effective for those who experience diarrhea as a primary symptom of IBS.

The Importance of Quality

There is a high degree of variability in probiotics. I prefer products that are proven to be shelf stable, meaning they do not have to be refrigerated. These probiotics are strong and hardy. Also, probiotics, even with the same name, are not always equal. For example, horses can be plow horses or Kentucky Derby winners, but technically, they are both horses. Some probiotics are stronger, more vigorous, and procreate more effectively. Make sure you are working with a company with a reputation for quality when you purchase probiotic supplements.

DOSAGE RECOMMENDATIONS

Taking a product with a large amount of probiotics is less important than making sure you get the right probiotics. My favorite probiotics are *Lactobacillus plantarum*, *Lactobacillus rhamnosus*, and *Bifidobacterium bifidum*. Start with at least 20 billion live, active cultures for best overall support.

Propolis:
Defender of the City

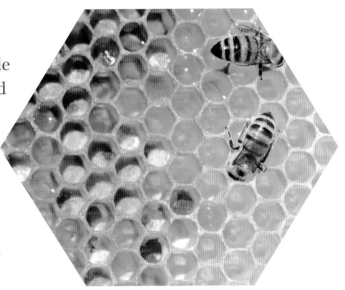

Ever wish you could see everything happening inside a beehive? If we could, we would certainly be amazed. We're all familiar with the bee's activity of making honey, but are you aware of another product of bees called propolis? It's time you knew more about this natural antibiotic, from our friends, the bees.

Propolis Seals the Deal

Bees gather resin, a liquid stored in the outer cells of trees and plants that oozes out when the tree is cut or injured and acts as a protection, much like blood clots in a wound. The bees modify the resin with their enzymes and processes the material by mixing it with beeswax. Next, they make it into a protective antibacterial glue and sealant to help keep the hive secure and safe from debris and predators. It makes perfect sense that the word "propolis" means "defender of the city" in Greek.

Propolis to the Rescue

Have you heard in the news how the over-prescribing of antibiotics has made bacterial infections very difficult to treat? This has led to resistant strains of *Staphylococcus aureus, E. coli, H. pylori,* and other dangerous bacteria. Researchers are finding out that propolis, especially the bioflavonoid-rich nutrients in extracts from controlled and managed bee populations is the answer. A study at the University of Heidelberg tested a proprietary propolis extract (GH2002) against a variety of disease-causing bacteria including MRSA and

Streptococcus pyogenes. Within six hours, propolis stopped the activity of *S. pyogenes,* the cause of strep throat and hard-to-stop skin infections. The study also found that it had a high degree of antibacterial activity against all tested MRSA strains, and inhibited candida.

Wide-Reaching Power

The power of propolis goes even further. Because it's rich in flavonoids, amino acids, and antioxidants it is also effective against two types of the herpes virus—HSV-1 and HSV-2. These are the viral infections that cause fever blisters (HSV-1) and genital herpes (HSV-2). With up to 90 percent of the population exposed to the virus that causes cold sores and fever blisters, propolis applied as a topical cream can be a great solution to the itching, burning, and tingling that signals an outbreak of the virus.

Propolis has also been found to have the ability to reduce cancer cells. A study done in Thailand suggests that propolis may be able to shrink both lung and cervical cancer cells after 24, 48, and 72 hours of treatment. These are just some of the examples using propolis as an antiviral, anti-inflammatory, and anti-tumor wonder of modern natural medicine. From daily use to ward off cold and flu, to use in fighting a tumor, to so many uses in between, you can count on propolis.

When it comes to propolis, "bee" selective and be healthy!

DOSAGE RECOMMENDATIONS

Make sure the propolis you choose clearly states that it contains no beeswax. In order to ensure a reliable form of propolis extract with consistent benefits, I recommend getting one that uses a GH2002 extract. Propolis in this supplement form is exclusively collected from carefully monitored hives in a defined area for controlled results. Start at 100 mg a day, and increase to one capsule twice daily for additional support. For cold sore and fever blister relief, choose a topical cream containing propolis, once again looking for the GH2002 extraction.

Pumpkin Seed Extract and the Prostate

Like so many of our most effective botanicals, pumpkin (*Cucurbita pepo*) has been used as food and medicine. Pumpkin species differ throughout the world, but many of them share common nutrients. While much of the research has been done on *Cucurbita pepo*, studies indicate that others are just as valuable.

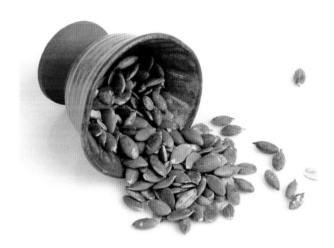

The seeds from this remarkable plant are naturally high in valuable minerals, including manganese, magnesium, copper, zinc, and iron. They also provide the amino acid tryptophan, antioxidant carotenoids, linoleic acid, and tocopherol, and are a good source of protein.

Beta-Sitosterol: A Major Component

For prostate health, one of the most valuable components of pumpkin seeds are phytosterols. Phytosterols have been described as the fat of plants, which I suppose is a pretty good comparison of their structure, generally, but doesn't quite encompass how valuable they are for our health. There are a lot of sources of phytosterols—flax, walnuts, and of course, pumpkin. Of the phytosterols, the one you're most likely to consume is beta-sitosterol.

Once absorbed in the digestive tract, beta-sitosterol is metabolized in the liver and travels to the other tissues in the body, including the prostate.

Benign prostate hyperplasia (BPH) is common for men because prostate enlargement is nothing unusual. The reason it affects the urinary flow is that the organ surrounds the urethra. So as it enlarges, it doesn't just grow outward, but inward, too—affecting the flow from the bladder to the urethra. When men feel like they have a slow stream, have to go often, or need to get up at night several times to go the bathroom, they may very likely be dealing with BPH.

However, if you have experienced urological problems and suspect it is BPH, you're not going to get enough of this valuable plant sterol through your diet alone. And this is where pumpkin seed extract can be especially helpful.

Makes BPH Symptoms Better

In scientific and clinical studies, pumpkin seed extract has been tested alone or in combination with other botanical ingredients. In these cases, the results have been remarkably consistent: pumpkin seed oils and extracts have reduced prostate volume and the symptoms of BPH, including overactive bladder and urinary incontinence.

For example, in a 12-month, randomized, double-blind, placebo-controlled study, men with BPH were already reporting a higher quality of life after only 3 months of using 320 mg of pumpkin seed oil. Those scores continued to improve by 6 months, as did urinary flow. Another group in the study, taking a combination of 320 mg of pumpkin seed oil and 320 mg of saw palmetto saw even stronger results, indicating a strong synergy between the two ingredients.

A multi-center clinical of over 2,000 men with BPH found that in only 12 weeks, pumpkin seed oil extract reduced urinary symptoms by 41 percent, and improved their quality of life by over 46 percent as rated in symptom score and questionnaires, respectively.

Other scientific research has shown a significant reduction in prostate weight and volume using pumpkin seed. It has also been found that pumpkin seed oil reduces the conversion of testosterone into a metabolite of the hormone called dihydrotestosterone, or DHT by inhibiting the action of an enzyme called 5-alpha reductase. As a byproduct of testosterone, too much DHT can cause a hormone imbalance that leads to prostate problems.

Bladder Improvement, Too

For men *and* women, bladder issues are a major concern as they get older. Often, overactive bladder or urinary urgency can simply be a matter of structure, strength, and capacity. In both women and men, bladder walls and the sphincter for the urinary tract (the valve that allows urine flow) can become weaker with age. This gives even small disruptions—a laugh, a sneeze—the potential to cause episodes of urinary leakage.

In a clinical study, pumpkin seed extract from *Cucurbita maxima*, the main species grown in Japan, was also shown to significantly relieve symptoms of urinary incontinence in men and women within just the first six weeks of the full 12-week trial.

Aside from alleviating prostate, bladder, and urinary issues, pumpkin seed oil may also be valuable for reducing blood pressure and promoting better pancreatic responses to high blood sugar.

Overall, pumpkin seed is one of the most effective natural medicines for men and women. It is safe and effective and is a smart choice for anyone dealing with incontinence, urgency, BPH, or other related health issues.

DOSAGE RECOMMENDATIONS

I would recommend a maintenance level of pumpkin seed extract at 500 mg daily.

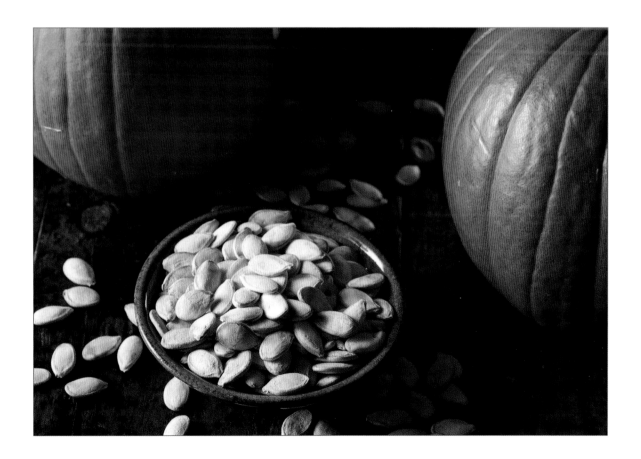

Ravintsara: Strong Immune Power

Ravintsara is a variety of *Cinnamomum camphora*, used in traditional medicine in Asia, but also introduced to Madagascar over 150 years ago. While the Asian varieties of this tree are used in traditional medicine and are naturally similar to the trees on Madagascar, the transplants have naturalized over time, as well. The difference in soil, growing conditions, and climate have given their oils a different chemical profile. In this case, ravintsara oil contains high levels of 1,8 cineole (giving it a scent much like eucalyptus) and has been shown to have strong antibacterial potential.

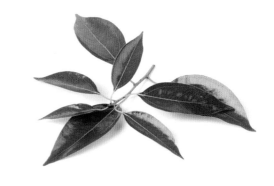

• •

Stronger than Bacteria

This makes ravintsara extremely valuable as an herbal intervention to deal with the problem of drug-resistant bacteria. Bacteria have become pretty tough over the past 50 years, due mostly to the overuse of prescription antibiotics and the current trend for antibacterial lotions and other health and beauty products. They have adapted and become resistant.

Of course, our lives leave us open to bacterial invasions all the time—travel, strange food and drink (especially on the road), crowded public spaces like shopping malls and airports, closed-in spaces with recirculated air like offices and airplanes, and of course, schools anytime they're in session. And certainly, you come into contact with bacteria every day. In fact, the surface of your desk at work may contain many times more bacteria than most bathrooms.

Because of the development of drug-resistant bacteria, researchers have investigated the mechanics of plant oils and their ability to prevent bacterial growth.

Cinnamomum camphora has been shown to inhibit *Streptococcus pyogenes,* the cause of strep throat and potentially life-threatening skin diseases.

Stops Inflammation and Protects Cells

Other scientific work has revealed that the botanical also inhibits breast tumor cells, and has anti-inflammatory actions (modulating cytokine, nitric oxide, and prostaglandin production) that account for its use in its original Asian variety for rheumatism, bronchitis, and general aches and pains.

But I think that the Madagascar variety of *Cinnamomum camphora*—ravintsara— may be even stronger for fighting colds and bacteria because of its much higher levels of 1,8 cineole.

Fights Colds without Side Effects

Plus, considering the high levels of inflammation involved in any kind of respiratory disease or condition, I believe that ravintsara is a definite must. And when you think about the side effects of common over-the-counter cold medicines, strong herbal essential oils make much more sense. They can get to the root of the problem and stop the causes *and* symptoms of colds.

DOSAGE RECOMMENDATIONS

A good dosage is 25–50 mg, two or three times daily. The best delivery system for ravintsara is in a base of extra virgin olive oil encapsulated in a softgel. I would avoid essential oils in canola or other unhealthy oils.

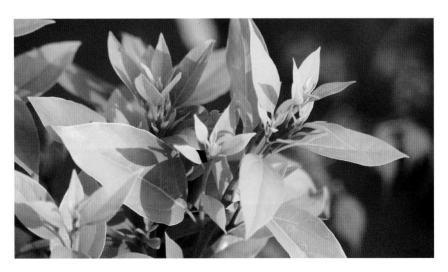

Rhodiola to the Rescue

A daptogens, including rhodiola, are a special group of herbs that do just as their name implies, help us to adapt. By definition, adaptogens must be non-toxic and restore balance to the body by working on all body systems. One of the largest uses today of rhodiola is to promote energy and vitality. Our energy reserves are constantly under attack, and in my opinion, virtually everyone could use more adaptogens in their daily routine.

. . . .

Adaptogens: From Surviving to Thriving

Rhodiola is an adaptogen that grows native in tundra-like areas of the world such as Northern Europe and Asia. Perhaps its ability to thrive in such harsh environments is a nice parallel to the benefits it bestows to us. While rhodiola has been used traditionally among the Vikings and Chinese emperors, it wasn't until about 50 years ago that the mechanisms of action and scientific validation came to light.

The Science of Stress

We know that stress can have numerous effects on the body: pain, fatigue, weakened immune system, obesity, and even heart disease. Fortunately, rhodiola has been clinically studied to help alleviate many of the common stress symptoms we see today. In a clinical study on stress-related fatigue, participants received rhodiola extract or placebo for 28 days. At the end of the study, the rhodiola group experienced significant reductions in fatigue and increased mental performance.

Rhodiola Reduces Inflammation

Inflammation and stress go hand-in-hand; if you can reduce one, chances are you can reduce the other. Rhodiola's effects were studied on a substance called C-reactive protein (CRP), which is associated with high levels of inflammation in the body. Rhodiola was shown to significantly decrease CRP in the study participants and this outcome lasted five days after the initial test period.

Alleviating Anxiety

Traditional uses for rhodiola include anxiety, depression, and other emotional imbalances. In a ten week study on generalized anxiety disorder (GAD), participants were given 340 mg of rhodiola per day. Participants were evaluated using the Hamilton Anxiety Rating Scale (HARS) and significant reductions occurred, which indicated an improvement in overall GAD symptoms.

Enhance Exercise Performance

Rhodiola has been favored by athletes and was even used by Russian Olympic contenders. Whether you're an aspiring Olympian, or just getting back into an exercise routine, rhodiola would be a great addition. Participants in a clinical study who took rhodiola for less than a week experienced significant increases in exercise ability, oxygen capacity, and elimination of carbon dioxide. Other studies have also confirmed rhodiola's ability to enhance endurance and help facilitate repair post-exercise.

Natural Cancer Killer

As if rhodiola's track record isn't impressive enough already, add anticancer properties to the list. A study on human colorectal cancer cells demonstrated rhodiola's ability to prevent cancer cell proliferation and promote cancer cell death. Similarly, a study on breast cancer cells also showed that rhodiola could prevent replication, cellular division, metastasis, and decrease certain inflammatory compounds. Rhodiola has also been shown to improve a condition called cachexia, the debilitating weight loss associated with many types of cancer.

Key Compounds

Whether you're looking for emotional support, extra endurance, inflammation reduction, cancer protection, or overall health improvement, rhodiola is a safe and effective natural medicine. There are many varieties of rhodiola, but I believe the most effective extracts come from *Rhodiola rosea*, which is clinically studied and standardized to contain rosavins and salidrosides. One clinically validated extract is called EPR-7. In a scientific study, EPR-7 was compared to seven other rhodiola extracts and found to be superior.

DOSAGE RECOMMENDATIONS

Many of the published human trials used dosages of 200–600 mg per day of rhodiola preparations that have consistent levels of these compounds. Rhodiola is often combined with other adaptogens like ashwagandha for even greater benefits. I recommend clinically studied EPR-7.

Saw Palmetto: Prostate Power

Saw Palmetto (*Serenoa repens*) is probably one of the best-studied botanicals for prostate enlargement. A small, low-growing plant with dark purple berries, it is found along the coast in Florida, Mississippi, and South Carolina.

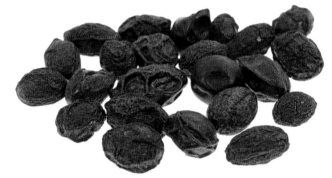

It is the berries of the saw palmetto plant that contain the compounds—including plant sterols and flavonoids—considered so important for reducing symptoms of benign prostate hyperplasia (BPH), and for inhibiting the risk of developing prostate cancer.

• • • • • • • • • • • • • • • • • • • •

Effects on Hormones

One of the reasons that saw palmetto is so well-regarded for prostate health is related to its ability to moderate hormone levels. Men's hormone levels change as they get older, and the result can be an enlarged prostate, commonly known as BPH. Because the prostate enlarges, it puts pressure on the urethra and causes problems including, a weak urinary stream, "stopping and starting" issues, and difficulty emptying the bladder.

While BPH is not the same as prostate cancer (nor does it mean you're going to get prostate cancer) it is interesting that saw palmetto studies show positive results inhibiting the effects of hormone conversion that cause BPH conditions and prostate growth.

A primary hormonal culprit in prostate enlargement is a derivative of testosterone called dihydrotestosterone, or "DHT." While it is normal for men's hormone balance to change over time and see an increase in DHT, too much can lead to prostate issues. The compounds in saw palmetto inhibit the enzyme 5-alpha reductase from metabolizing high levels of testosterone into DHT. Saw palmetto also prevents the binding of

DHT to androgenic receptors, which can lead to enlargement of the prostate as well.

Additionally, saw palmetto extract has a mild anti-inflammatory ability, blocking COX-2 and, to an extent, 5-LOX pathways. Not only does this help reduce some the swelling of the prostate, but it also fights the inevitable cellular damage that occurs *because* of inflammation. Clinical studies and scientific research has examined the effectiveness of saw palmetto, both on its own and combined with other ingredients.

Clinical Research

A common way of testing the effectiveness of medicines for the prostate is the International Prostate Symptom Score, which measures diagnostic questions, including urinary frequency, bladder emptying, and urgency. Combined with that, many clinical tests also ask individuals quality of life questions to gather real world information about how people actually feel a specific treatment is affecting their lives.

One clinical study was a year-long trial involving 47 men with BPH with an average age of 53. In just three months, the groups taking saw palmetto alone or combined with pumpkin seed oil—another strong ingredient for prostate concerns—noted a reduction in their overall symptom score and an improvement in their quality of life. Over the course of the study, the maximal urinary flow for men taking saw palmetto improved as well (as it did in the pumpkin seed group.) That means that a commonly-available herbal ingredient helped stop

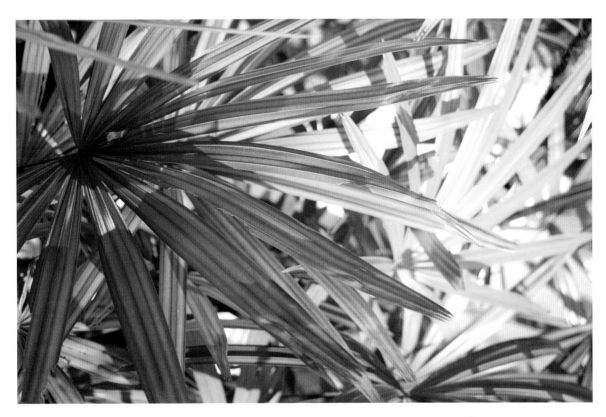

that "need to go" feeling that is so common to men—even after they've just been to the restroom. This is very positive news for men looking for relief from symptoms of BPH without worrying about the side effects of synthetic drugs.

Another placebo-controlled clinical study of men 45 and older found similar results for urinary tract symptoms in six months, and a study using a combination of saw palmetto and nettle root (*Urtica dioica*) extract showed the same efficacy as finasteride, a common drug for BPH, but with better tolerance and fewer side effects.

In fact, there are a number of clinical trials and reviews that suggest a combination of saw palmetto with other nutrients are highly effective, and that may be an excellent option if you're concerned about BPH or are at risk of prostate cancer. For some, the combined strength of botanical compounds, vitamin co-factors, or minerals can work more effectively than one alone. It all depends on an individual's response.

Safe and Effective

Overall, a review of the most important clinical studies and scientific literature found that most of the published trials truly show that saw palmetto significantly improved urinary flow in men with BPH. It also acknowledged that saw palmetto works on many fronts—as an anti-inflammatory, anti-androgenic (hormone balancing), and an anti-proliferative effect, important for keeping prostate growth in check.

But whether used as a single herbal ingredient or as part of a combination, saw palmetto has a lot to offer. But ultimately, for men moving through adult life, starting a regimen of this powerful botanical may be one of the best preventive steps available.

DOSAGE RECOMMENDATIONS

As a single herbal ingredient, a total level of 320 mg twice daily is the right range. As part of a combination of nutrients for the prostate, it will work synergistically, so less may be required.

Schisandra: Endurance, Strength, and Resilience

Native to China, schisandra (*Schisandra chinensis*) is a woody vine that bears clusters of tiny, bright red berries. The berries are called "Wu Wei Zi" in Chinese, which translates to "five-flavor fruit," based on their salty, sweet, sour, pungent, and bitter flavors. Like ashwagandha and rhodiola, schisandra is an adaptogen, which means it's a type of herb that helps the body deal with psychological and physical stressors and adapt to the environment around it. Schisandra, in particular, has been used traditionally for millennia to slow the aging process, improve concentration, fight fatigue, and enhance immune function.

Promotes Endurance and Reduces Stress

Schisandra is a potent general tonic that can decrease fatigue, enhance physical performance, and promote endurance. While the mechanism of action of schisandra is not completely understood, beneficial compounds called lignans found in the seeds of the berry may be responsible. Schisandra counters stress by reducing the levels of stress hormones in the blood. It also has strong anti-inflammatory and antioxidant properties.

Enhances Concentration

Several human clinical studies show that schisandra improves concentration, coordination, and endurance. Much like rhodiola, schisandra helps to prevent mental fatigue and increases accuracy and quality of work. In various human clinical studies with people who definitely need to be able to function under stress and lack of sleep, including soldiers, doctors, students, and other groups, schisandra demonstrated superior benefits and helped keep everyone focused.

Protects the Liver

Schisandra is also known to improve digestive health, increase enzyme production, and help protect and cleanse the liver. Since the liver is responsible for removing toxins from the body, it is crucial to your overall health and plays a significant role in immune system function, as well. In a Chinese study of 40 people, schisandra was shown to increase antioxidant activity, improve liver function, and provide relief from fatty liver disease. The participants also experienced an increase in glutathione, which is an essential "master" antioxidant for overall health.

What to Look For

When choosing an effective supplement, make sure to look for one that contains schisandra that has been standardized for one type of lignan in particular—schizandrin. This type of lignan will provide you with the optimal potency and benefits from the herb.

DOSAGE RECOMMENDATIONS

An effective dosage for schisandra is approximately 500 mg, one to three times daily.

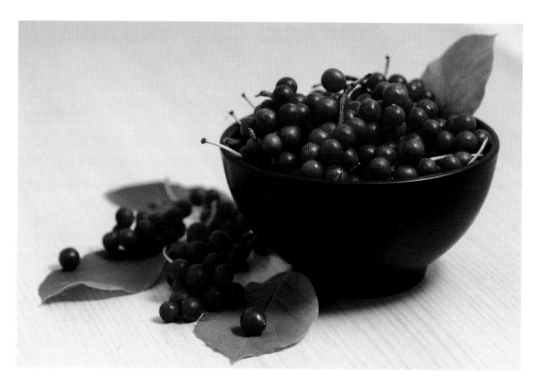

Sea Buckthorn: Master of Moisture

When you hear about omega fatty acids, omega-3 probably comes to mind first. But you may not know that there are a range of other omega fatty acids with excellent health benefits. One in particular is omega-7, which is extremely useful for healthy skin, heart problems, dry eyes, and more. Omega-7 is found in just a few foods, with one of the richest sources being the pulp of the Sea Buckthorn berry. This berry is often referred to as a "nutrient bomb" and contains more than 200 bioactive compounds including natural vitamins, antioxidants, essential fatty acids, and plant sterols. Omega-7 fatty acids are incorporated into the walls of your cells and help the cells better hold on to moisture.

• •

Makes Skin Look Younger

The aging process considerably alters the skin, making it less elastic and increasing the appearance of wrinkles and fine lines. It can be accelerated by poor nutrition, lack of sleep, excessive sun exposure, environmental toxins, and stress. Sea buckthorn oil protects skin from oxidative damage and restores skin moisture and elasticity. It is also an excellent source of essential nutrients for regulating moisture and sensitivity of skin.

In a clinical study, healthy women with an average age of 61 years took sea buckthorn oil or a placebo for three months. Those using sea buckthorn saw a 49 percent improvement in skin moisture (33 percent in just one month) and a 9.2 percent improvement in wrinkle depth, meaning skin wrinkles were less severe. The extra hydration provided by the sea buckthorn actually works to smooth out the skin. This same study also showed a 26 percent improvement in skin elasticity.

Essentially, sea buckthorn oil slows down the aging process of the skin. It is also the perfect natural solution for anyone dealing with atopic eczema or dermatitis, and promotes wound healing, too.

Protects the Heart and Cardiovascular System

The effect of sea buckthorn oil on cardiovascular health has been widely studied. Results prove sea buckthorn's ability to improve blood lipid profiles and reduce risk factors for cardiovascular disease. It also increases the level of good cholesterol, reduces the harmful effects of bad cholesterol, and acts on platelet aggregation to prevent the formation of harmful blood clots.

Relieves Dry Eyes and Soothes Mucous Membranes

The nutrients in sea buckthorn work together to keep the body's mucous membranes, including the tear film of the eyes and sensitive vaginal tissue, moist and strong. It's actually extremely effective for those suffering from Sjögren's syndrome, an autoimmune disease that causes inflammation and dryness in the mouth, tear glands, lining of the bronchial airways, and vagina.

In a placebo-controlled, double-blind, crossover study, patients with Sjögren's syndrome used either sea buckthorn oil or a placebo for three months. Those in the sea buckthorn group showed greater improvement in vaginal mucosa and overall symptom relief, including burning, itching, pain, secretion, and dryness—including dry eyes and mouth.

The Best Sea Buckthorn

When you look for a sea buckthorn supplement, make sure the extract you find is rich in many nutrients, including omega-7, but also omega-3, 6, and 9. Plus, a complete sea buckthorn oil extract includes phytosterols, tocopherols, and carotenoids, just like the material used in the studies. My personal favorite sea buckthorn is a combination of the extract of the sea buckthorn berry *and* seed oil combinations in a proprietary ratio. It is the most clinically studied sea buckthorn product in the world.

DOSAGE RECOMMENDATIONS

To support the hydration of eyes, skin, heart, and other mucous membranes throughout the body, supplement with 500 mg of sea buckthorn daily. For advanced support, it is perfectly safe to increase your daily dosage to 1,000 mg to 3,000 mg.

Silica: Move Over Calcium— Silica for Bones!

Our bones are a complex, living system and need certain nutrients for optimal functioning. When we think of building bones, calcium always comes to mind, but there is another mineral that is absolutely necessary for strong bones: silica. Silica helps to oversee the bone-building process by bringing more calcium into the bone matrix and holding it there. Scientific research shows it can even improve calcium absorption into the bones by 50 percent. Even better, silica helps to prevent calcium from leaving the bones. This is great news for anyone struggling with bone density issues, like osteopenia or osteoporosis.

• •

Silica Connects the Body

Silica helps to form collagen, which is the main protein in the body. We need collagen to form the structures that literally hold us together—tendons, ligaments, bone, cartilage, and blood vessels. Collagen lays down the framework for calcium to build upon and gives our bones flexibility and strength. During a twelve-month clinical study, 65 women experienced significant decreases in the amount of minerals that were resorbed, or moved out of their bones.

So without silica, our bodies wouldn't be able to create collagen, and our bones would not hold together. Collagen is also necessary for our skin, nails, and hair, and has been used in France to promote youth and diminish the signs of aging. The aging process decreases our natural production of collagen and causes our skin to lose elasticity. By adding silica into your supplement regimen, the body can produce more consistent levels of collagen throughout any stage of life.

Our Brains Need Silica

There is emerging evidence that silica may be beneficial for people struggling with neurological issues, like Alzheimer's disease. When we consume certain metals, such as aluminum, if they are not excreted properly, these harmful substances can migrate to our brain. An overabundance of heavy metals can cause increased levels of inflammation, cellular death, prevent proper cellular communication, and alter our gene expression. A 2013 study demonstrated that drinking silica-rich mineral water for twelve weeks was able to increase the amount of aluminum expelled by the body. Some of the participants even experienced improvements in their thinking and cognitive performance. Additionally, a separate study found that increasing silica intake by 10 mg per day could significantly reduce the risk of dementia. Silica is very promising for neurological health and the aging process in general.

Smile with Silica

Another interesting use for silica is in dentistry. Because silica helps to form the body's glue—collagen—it strengthens the connection between our jaws and teeth. A study involving patients receiving dental implants demonstrated that silica helped to heal the surrounding tissues and stabilize the jawbone during surgery. Plus, out of the 37 participants involved, none experienced implant loss.

Selecting the Best Silica

Silica can be difficult to absorb and factors like aging and hormonal issues, including hypothyroidism, can greatly decrease silica's absorption. My favorite form of silica comes from the above-ground portions of the spring horsetail (*Equisetum arvense*) plant. This special silica is clinically studied and part of a complex that includes marine oils to enhance absorption.

DOSAGE RECOMMENDATIONS

For optimal health, I think 20–40 mg per day of this unique silica is necessary. However, you can certainly temporarily increase this to 60 mg a day if you have a fracture.

St. John's Wort: Effective for Depression

Did you realize that in the United States, an average of *16 million adults suffer from depression?* Those who seek help often end up on a roller coaster of prescription medications, which can cause other problems like weight gain, sluggishness, sexual problems, fatigue, and even worsening of depression. These sad facts could be different if people would turn to a natural solution—St. John's wort.

• •

Problems with the Pills

The biochemistry behind depression is extremely complicated and elusive. One medication after another tries to inhibit the breakdown of specific neurotransmitters needed to function properly. These drugs focus solely on communication signals in the brain while trying to restore chemical signals, which are minimized by this disease. At the same time, the very drugs meant to help with depression cause multiple side effects. This initiates a switch to yet another drug, and the same problems start all over again.

A Bum Buzz

In multiple studies, St. John's wort (*Hypericum perforatum*) has exhibited an extraordinary ability to alleviate depression. Still, you may have heard buzz about this wonderful herb not always living up to its promise. The problem was never the St. John's, but rather irregular dosing and lack of standardization to the most beneficial compound in the plant. Fortunately, a special 900 mg once-daily St. John's wort extract available that can remain in the bloodstream for up to 24 hours or more. Taken consistently, it can stop depression and dysthymia, reduce anxieties and fear, boost positive natural brain chemistry, and help anyone suffering depression to feel hopeful again.

Proof Upon Proof

There's a vast array of convincing studies on St. John's wort. Do some research on your own, and you'll be amazed at how it compares to prescription medication for depression. For example, in one randomized, double-blind, 6-week study comparing St. John's wort to fluoxetine (commonly marketed as Prozac) the botanical was found to be just as effective as the drug. Also, St. John's wort's safety was found to be substantially superior to fluoxetine. Those taking fluoxetine reported agitation, dizziness, tiredness, anxiety, and erectile dysfunction. When looking at the data from 29 clinical trials that included 18 placebo comparisons and 17 comparisons with standard antidepressant drugs the conclusions said it all. St. John's wort was consistently superior compared to placebo, and "similarly effective as standard antidepressants"—but with fewer noted side effects. But, remember—you need a consistent, 900 mg amount each day. I believe St. John's wort is one of the premier natural medicines and should be a first-line of defense to help you feel vibrant, healthy, and happy again.

DOSAGE RECOMMENDATION

An optimal dose is 900 mg each day. Using a once-a-day specially formulated tablet replaces the need to take multiple doses throughout the day.

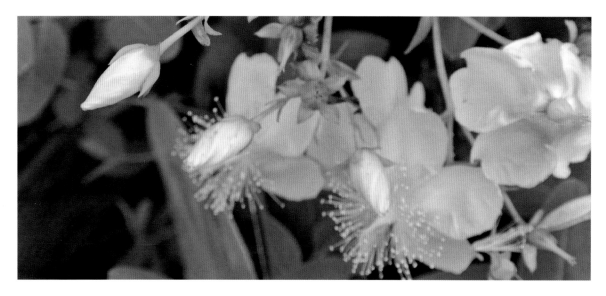

White Willow Bark: Especially Good for Back Pain

What do you think Native Americans and early settlers turned to when they had back pain or a fever? They turned to the bark of the white willow tree for answers. Also used for centuries in China as a natural pain reliever, white willow bark still holds answers for those suffering from pain, today.

• •

From a Tea to a Pill

Ancient civilizations and native groups made a tea of white willow bark for pain. Even Hippocrates, the father of modern medicine, promoted the tea's use to reduce fever and alleviate pain. In 1828, European chemists isolated a compound from willow extract and named it "salicin" after the genus of the willow tree, *Salix*. A decade later, another potent compound was found called salicylic acid. Once the molecular formula of salicylic acid was decoded, it could be turned into a synthetic form called acetylsalicylic acid that was faster and cheaper to produce. Aspirin was born, and white willow extract fell off the radar.

Back to Nature's Aspirin

With the side effects that can come from aspirin, including stomach bleeding, researchers have turned back to the original natural compound. They are relying once again on the salicin from white willow bark that is responsible for lowering prosta-glandins, the hormone-like compounds in the body that can cause inflammation, aches, and pains. In one clinical trial, white willow equaled the pain relief of the prescription drug Vioxx. This non-steroidal anti-inflammatory drug (NSAID) is no longer on the market because of harmful side effects. However, this study shows the power of white willow bark extract to provide pain relief without dangerous side effects. In another trial, white willow bark reduced pain by 14 percent compared to the placebo group, which experienced a two percent *increase* in pain.

Safe Pain Reduction

Research continues to prove that white willow bark is a safe anti-inflammatory for chronic lower back pain, joint problems, and osteoarthritis compared to other NSAIDs, including aspirin. While white willow bark can be used alone, I believe that its synergistic strength when combined with other ingredients like devil's claw, boswellia, curcumin, and DLPA, is a very effective answer for inflammation relief and back pain. Make sure when getting a white willow bark extract by itself or in conjunction with some other strong herbal pain fighters that you look for one that is standardized for at least 15 percent salicin, its primary pain-fighting compound. It's a wonderful weapon to have in your arsenal to fight pain.

DOSAGE RECOMMENDATIONS

Look for white willow bark standardized for at least 15 percent salicin. A typical dose is 120–240 mg a day.

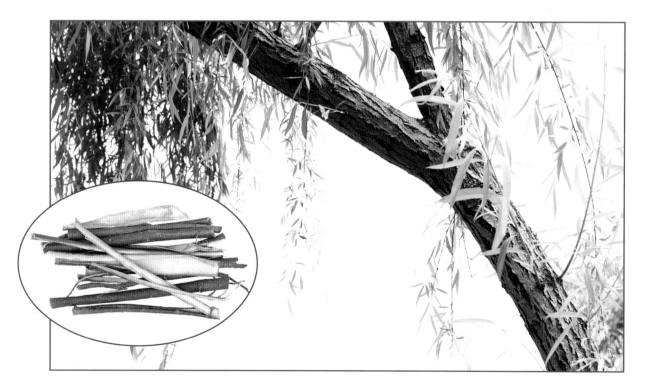

Diet for a Long Life

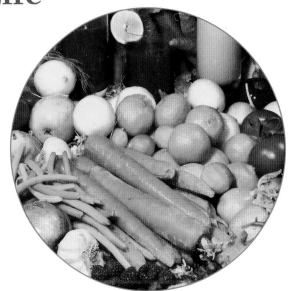

Want to live a long, healthy life and achieve a healthy weight in the process? Eat heartily and make sure you get plenty of animal protein and good healthy fats in your diet. It's true. And that story you've been told about cholesterol being bad for you? Forget all about it.

• •

In fact, if you're over the age of 48, stop worrying about cholesterol levels completely. The people who have told you to stop eating red meat, butter, eggs, and other nutritionally vital whole foods are just flat out wrong. So where did this idea come from?

As it turns out, this idea came from research centered on rabbits.

What happened is this: researchers fed large quantities of oxidized and purified cholesterol to rabbits, who not surprisingly, suffered severe damage to their hearts and arteries.

Of course there's one problem. Rabbits eat grass and plants.

They don't consume foods with cholesterol and don't naturally have any mechanism to handle and control cholesterol.

However, we do.

It's amazing that researchers used rabbits—and this experiment's evidence—to try to understand a human's requirement for animal fats and cholesterol and their mechanism of action. So the new low fat diet was born with no scientific evidence that it prevents heart disease or strokes. And this has been a health disaster ever since.

If you just look back to the kinds of diets that our grandparents and great-grandparents ate 60 to 80 years ago, according to today's modern medical beliefs, *everyone* should have been overweight. And you know that's not true. Even a casual glance at older photographs or old movies shows how much thinner people were in the past compared to where we are now with our high carbohydrate diets mistakenly recommended by medical experts in the interest of avoiding fats. Granted, a big part of that was the availability of food—no surplus of vending machines and snack foods—and the fact that people weren't generally as sedentary as we've become.

But our abundance has come with a severe price. The emphasis our diets have on refined carbs and sugar hasn't just resulted in people being overweight and out of shape, but being sick and exhausted all of the time, experiencing high blood pressure and the explosion of type 2 diabetes.

It's not surprising. Without animal proteins and fats, the body doesn't get the nutrients it needs to survive and thrive. Whole foods and whole fats are what we are supposed to be eating—that's why people generally feel so hungry when they try to get by on processed, refined, and "lite" diets—they're facing a huge nutritional deficit.

According to the Centers for Disease Control (CDC), obesity rates are at least 25 percent or more in 34 states—and in 25 of those the rate is over 30 percent. So far, no statistical reversal of this trend is on the horizon. How could it be, when we've been told so often that perfectly healthy, wholesome, life-enhancing foods are the enemy?

There's a much better way to eat that satisfies our nutritional needs and our taste buds. It centers on real, whole traditional foods that were the mainstay in the early 1900s. The diet of our ancestors, a traditional diet (or very similar to a ketogenic diet), was high in all the vitamins and minerals and satisfied our appetite.

But today, because foods are refined, processed, and stripped of nutrients, they convert to sugar at a high rate. This causes us to eat more and in turn, secrete more insulin, which then causes the body to produce and store more fat. Therefore, it is not fat that makes you fat; it is carbohydrates that make you fat.

The traditional and ketogenic diets simply replicate much of what humanity ate for breakfast, lunch and dinner for two million years. Needless to say, there was not a lot of processing going on. They include a *lot* of animal protein (which most likely helped our brains grow and adapt), high animal fat, green, leafy plants, and low carbohydrates.

After all, our original diet was approximately 30 percent animal protein, 60 percent animal fat, and 10 percent *non-starchy* carbohydrates primarily from fruits and vegetables, so it makes sense to return to this ratio.

And because of that, giving up refined grain-and-sugar based carbohydrates is an absolute must. Once you make that switch, you'll stop weight gain, insulin resistance, and inflammation. If you're used to carbs, letting them go can be tough, no doubt about it. But with discipline and gradually seeing healthy benefits, you'll be amazed how easy it can be to adopt a new diet. My bottom line: consume no more than 72 grams of carbohydrates daily.

Does all of this sound challenging? It can be. But the results are worth it and it's an extremely satisfying way to eat. Consider the delicious foods you can enjoy on this diet: grass-fed beef, bison, poultry, butter, whole fat cheese, nuts, whole fat dairy products, vegetables, berries of all kinds, eggs, fish, olive oil, and coconut oil—to name just a few. Believe me, whatever you choose from this diet is definitely going to keep you fueled and healthy much better than the trans-fat and refined grain-and-sugar foods you may have been following in the past.

PROTEINS EVERY DAY

Proteins are our original energy and power foods and they are absolutely necessary to maintain a strong body. I'd like to share my favorite food sources for great protein, and why they should definitely be a part of your diet. Remember that animal protein is rich in readily-absorbable amino acids, which are the building blocks of the body and mind.

Must-Have Proteins:

- Grass-fed beef
- Bison
- Elk
- Venison
- Lamb
- Rabbit
- Poultry
- Salmon
- Eggs
- Nuts

AN ABUNDANCE OF HEALTHY FATS

The fear of fat has led to an epidemic of diseases that have occurred primarily because we have *reversed* the ratio of our food groups from high animal proteins/animal fats and low carbohydrates, to high refined carbohydrates and sugar and little or no healthy animal protein and animal fats. In fact, many Americans probably consume around 60 to 70 percent of their meals as carbohydrates (mostly refined and processed), and 20 to 30 percent *unhealthy* fats (omega-6 from vegetable oils, shortening and margarine) and only 10 percent from protein.

Those highly processed foods that advertise as being non-fat, low fat, and two-percent fat actually contain hydrogenated fats and trans-fatty acids—the *real* contributors to cancer and heart disease. The omega-6 fatty acid group found in soybean, corn, safflower, canola and other unhealthy oils *greatly* exceeds the ratio of the much healthier, natural omega-3 fatty acids and they are not balanced by other fatty acids in any way that is truly healthy.

The processed fats known as "trans fats" are especially dangerous. These processed fats have been changed—hydrogenated—to make fully or "partially hydrogenated" trans-fat. Hydrogenation is a chemical process in which hydrogen atoms are added to a *liquid* vegetable fat to change it to a *solid*—margarine being a prime example. Thank goodness we're getting smarter about trans fats and making progress in eliminating them from foods.

In Denmark, where it has been illegal for foods to contain more than two percent trans fats since 2004, deaths from heart disease have dropped by 20 percent. This seems to make sense when you consider that the 2006 review found that with a two percent increase of calories consumed as trans fat, the incidence of coronary heart disease increased by 23 percent.

Additionally, trans fats can raise total cholesterol levels and deplete good cholesterol (HDL), which helps protect against heart disease. By contrast—and probably a surprise for many—saturated fats do *not* deplete HDL—in fact, they may even increase it.

Science appears to be catching up to the idea that fats and animal proteins aren't bad for you. In the meantime, I'd suggest you adjust your diet accordingly, and enjoy the benefits and taste of real food.

Must-Have Fats in Your Diet

- ☒ Cream and Butter
- ☒ Raw milk from goats or cows— but skip processed milk
- ☒ Lard
- ☒ Coconut oil
- ☒ Olive oil
- ☒ Sesame oil
- ☒ Avocado oil

NUTRIENT-RICH FRUITS AND VEGETABLES

Choose colorful fruits and vegetables because that indicates they have a high antioxidant value. Berries, for example, have compounds called anthocyanins, a type of flavonoid that provides extremely potent antioxidant activity, protecting cells from the harmful effects of oxidation and the inflammation that often follows.

Eat a variety of fruits and vegetables each day, because they provide so many valuable nutrients. Getting the amount you need really isn't as difficult as you may think. After all, a serving of grapes, blueberries, and carrots is just one cup, and even one small apple counts as a serving.

Must-Have Fruits and vegetables

- ☒ Apples
- ☒ Asparagus
- ☒ Blueberries
- ☒ Carrots
- ☒ Cherries
- ☒ Cruciferous family: broccoli, cauliflower, Brussels sprouts
- ☒ Garlic
- ☒ Grapes
- ☒ Onions
- ☒ Pomegranate
- ☒ Spinach and other greens
- ☒ Sweet Potatoes (sparingly)

BEGIN EATING A TRADITIONAL DIET

As you start switching over to a traditional or a ketogenic diet, remember to plan your meals. It'll stop you from being tempted to go to fast food or processed options that are laden with nitrates, sodium, and trans-fatty acids. There is no reason you can't feel fantastic. Just remember healthy fats do not cause weight gain, excessive carbohydrates cause weight gain. And in the United States, most of the carbs we eat are so refined that they do us no good at all nutritionally—they only spike our blood sugar levels and add unhealthy weight.

The Benefits

- ☒ Stop sugar cravings and weight gain

- ☒ Eliminate brain fog and fatigue

- ☒ Prevent or reverse diabetes

- ☒ Reduce inflammation and joint pain

- ☒ Slow progression of Parkinson's and Alzheimer's diseases

- ☒ Stop oxidative stress and damage to the cells

After just a short time, you'll notice a difference. I can guarantee you that you'll have more energy, a trimmer body, a better waistline, and feel more vibrant and healthy overall.

Love Your Exercise (And Don't Spend Too Much Time On It)

I think there is a lot of misinformation about exercise out there. Many people are led to believe that it either takes too much time (I can't schedule a three mile run each day) or money (gym memberships are too expensive for my budget) to get into shape and be healthy. Or, they figure that if they can't look like a supermodel in a short time, they might as well not bother.

• •

But all of these are wrong-minded ideas. You don't need a surplus of time or money to get in shape, and not even supermodels look like supermodels without the air-brushing. All you need is commitment and maybe 20 minutes set aside for exercise about three times a week.

There was a time when I had an intensive workout regimen that was very close to what I'd call the typical exercise plan. I had a program of running for cardiovascular conditioning, plus additional weight lifting. I was doing about one to one and a half hours, three to four times a week.

It was beneficial exercise, but just too time consuming. With my busy schedule of running a business, having a family, and extensive travel, I found that I just could not afford the time I was devoting

to working out. I'm sure that's a familiar situation for many people.

But there's a better way to exercise that gets results and doesn't weigh down your schedule.

Short-burst Exercise: Kettlebells

In my search for a shorter, but still effective, exercise program, I ran across information on kettlebell training. If you've never seen a kettlebell, it looks like a cannonball with a handle and weighs anywhere from five to 106 pounds. My goal was to give my 400+ muscles, including the most important muscle, my heart, a vigorous workout in the shortest period of time. I kept seeing mention of an exercise program designed by Dr. Al Sears called PACE. A good friend,

Dr. Jonathan Wright, also made me aware of it. My routine is similar to the one Dr. Sears advocates, because I could not afford the time to work on individual muscle groups but still wanted to stay reasonably healthy, lean, and toned. I started working out on my own with kettlebells. My routine lasted 12–20 minutes, two or three times a week.

Over the course of two years, I was able to stay in very good shape and did not lose the benefits of my prior exercise routine. It was proof that I could stay as fit as before, but in a fraction of the time. Everybody can do this routine. You select the type of exercise and the degree of intensity. Combine that with rest in between the exercises, and you have the program.

In my 12–20 minute exercise program, I primarily use a series of kettlebell swings and a stationary recumbent bike. I use either a 44 pound or 53 pound kettlebell and do a kettlebell swing 30–35 times, which takes about 60 seconds and is like running 100 to 200 yards as fast as you can.

I then do a two-minute rest (active) following the intense burst of activity. My two minutes of rest is usually at the lowest level on a recumbent bike. I call this active rest. This is to provide continued circulation of the blood and to remove lactic acid from the muscles.

Depending on your level of fitness, you can start with a five-pound kettlebell or whatever is most suitable. Work your way up to the weight that gives you the best workout.

KETTLEBELL SWINGS

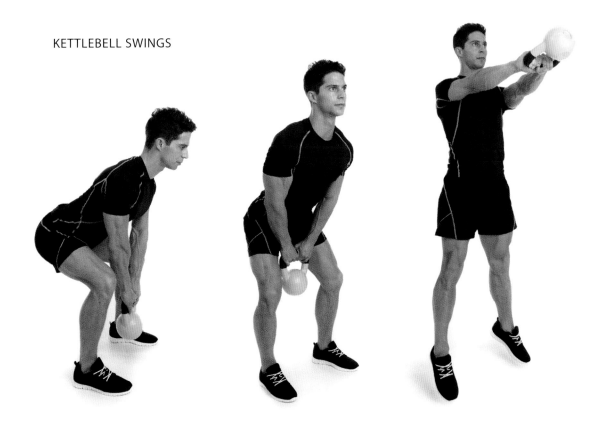

1. **Kettlebell swings:** 60 seconds to full exertion

2. **Active rest:** two minutes (walking, stationary bike, etc.)

3. **Repeat** sequence of exertion and active rest for 12–20 minutes

Even if you can only begin exercising and doing kettlebell swings using a five-pound weight, that would be a good place to start and progressively increase your intensity. You want to continue doing the swing until you run out of breath and then take a two-minute active rest. Repeat this sequence five or six times or as long as it takes to do in a period of 12–20 minutes. Some people do the kettlebell swing for 30–35 swings, and then for their rest period they jump rope for two minutes. I can't for the life of me jump rope so I use the recumbent bike as an active rest period. It is never a good idea to sit down for your rest period. You want to continue moving. You can even just walk around or bounce on your feet.

When the kettlebell swing is done correctly and over a sufficient period of time, every muscle in the body is working. It's not a squat, it's a hinge movement. If you make it into a squat exercise, you will put too much stress on your back. (See the resources listed at the end of this article for instructions.) The whole idea is to exercise for 40 to 60 seconds with a two-minute rest and repeat this cycle three to six times at your highest level of intensity. You can review my video on training at www.terrytalksnutrition.com/health-articles/terrys-exercise-plan/.

The Farmer's Walk

Another intensive, but short-burst workout I've incorporated into my regimen is called the farmer's walk. This form of exercise is exceptionally simple and it's based on how farmers in the past would commonly carry two pails of milk or two milk cans, one in each hand. To mimic this loaded carry, pick up two equal weights, one in each hand, they could be dumbbells, kettle bells, or two pails equally filled with salt or sand. This type of loaded carry is a great way to build on your core muscles in your trunk, keep your sense of balance finely tuned, and develop long-term strength and endurance.

Posture is extremely important in exercise, and a loaded carry like the farmer's walk is no exception. Maintain your posture and keeping your back straight helps develop the muscles in your shoulders, lower back, and upper arms. It also evenly distributes the weight along your thighs and calf muscles. In fact, done properly, the farmer's walk can build and tone virtually every muscle group.

Here's what you can do:

℘ Start off with a weight that is relatively heavy for you. Don't try to compete with the weight used by someone else, but carry a weight that challenges you for two methods of working out. One method is to carry a very heavy weight equally in each hand and walk for 20 to 40 yards or further if you can, probably until your grip gives out and stop, catch your breath, and return to your starting position. Repeat this cycle two or three times. Another method is to use a lighter weight, but maybe walk for 100 or 200 yards.

☒ You may walk a circuit in your yard, gym, or down your driveway for as long as you are able to maintain a good upright posture. For example, if you have the space, walk for about 20 yards (or whatever is the longest section of your backyard) back and forth.

☒ Then catch your breath and rest for a minute or two.

Coach Dan John has used this method of training and considered it to be a game changer. You will notice body changes and strength in a matter of three weeks when executing the farmer's walk two or three times a week. In fact, Dan believes the farmer's walk is the only exercise you need to do if you have limited time to exercise. You can find more on farmer's walk at danjohn.net, or at romanfitnesssystems.com/articles/loaded-carries/.

Choose Something that You Love

If kettlebells or the farmer's walk don't seem like your preferred forms of exercise, that's okay—choose something that you love and stick with it.

Choosing an activity that you enjoy means that you'll want to stick with it. Consider any of these, or even factor in your time spent gardening, doing yard work, or simply running errands. Keeping track of your daily steps or activities with a popular app or a pedometer can be a fun

way of gauging your progress, too. Here are a few ideas—and no matter how fun they are—they all count toward keeping you healthy. In fact, I think that the less you consider exercise to be a chore and the more it simply becomes a part of your life, the more you'll wonder how you ever got along being sedentary.

☒ Walking

☒ Swimming

☒ Bicycling

☒ Hiking or climbing

☒ Dancing

☒ Playing physical games with friends (basketball, soccer, etc)

☒ Yoga or Pilates

Simply pick something that works with your schedule and don't worry about putting in long hours at the gym.

There's good solid evidence that short-burst exercise works.

Consider this well-cited study by researchers at Laval University in Quebec. They divided participants into two groups, a long duration exercise group and an interval short term exercise group. The long duration group cycled continuously for up to 45 minutes. The short term group cycled for bursts of 15 to 90 minutes and rested in between sets.

Not surprisingly, the duration group burned twice the calories, so you'd think they'd burn more fat, right? They didn't. When the researchers recorded body composition measurements between the two groups, the *interval* group—exercising in small bursts—lost the most fat. Nine times more, in fact, for every calorie burned.

The best thing is that you don't have to be a trained athlete to see results. Researchers at the University of Guelph found that for untrained active adults, about 18 hours of high-intensity interval exercise over the course of six weeks (one hour, three days a week) increased the ability of their muscles to burn fat and carbohydrates.

High-intensity exercise begets better exercise and better muscle tone and recovery, too. In some cases, just two weeks of high-intensity training was similar to two weeks of endurance training. It has also shown the same benefits for metabolism and cardiovascular health, even though the individuals spent up to 90 percent less time exercising.

Like so many things in life, moderation is a key here. If you've been sedentary for a while and feel like a bit of a couch potato, don't plunge in and do the maximum level of exercise right off the bat. You may feel enthusiastic at first, but you could also be setting yourself up for unnecessary muscle soreness, injury, and frustration. When people start off being too zealous about their new workout regimen, it can be easy to get overwhelmed and quit, taking an all or nothing approach.

But you deserve to tailor a workout regimen that you can *consistently* perform. And that's the key. Keep at it, and make it part of your life. If you exercise regularly, you can add years to your life and make a noticeable difference in your physical and mental well-being.

If you want to stay in shape, regular exercise is a must. The type of exercise, consistency, and the time you ultimately put in overall matters most. For example, if you like cycling, go as fast as you can, as far as you can for 12 to 20 minutes. If you like running, sprint in short bursts for 200 meters. Whatever you choose, set the stopwatch or timer on your phone and stick with it. You'll probably be surprised at how quickly the time passes, and how little time is really required for a great workout.

Aside from the obvious physical benefits, regular exercise exerts a powerful positive effect on your mind. Making it a positive habit will help evaporate your tension and worries, and help you feel better overall. It's simply one of the best natural medicines in the world.

The End of the Book, But the Beginning of Your New Life

Hello Friends,

I'm so glad we've been able to connect through this book. It was a labor of love, dedicated to the goal of making a difference in your life and the lives of those you care about. There's one more vitamin I need to talk about, and it's one that is not mentioned that often.

That's Vitamin YOU!

All the knowledge contained in this book is worthless for you unless you take it and apply it to your life. That being said, here are a few more tips to make sure you are getting the very best that these nutrients have to offer—so that you can get the benefit of what they bring to create a more vibrant life.

- **Become a fan of research and clinical studies.** You don't need to be a scientist to explore clinical studies on herbs and vitamins. Make sure the supplements you take have sound clinical science behind them. Doing research on the web at such sites as pubmed.gov and talking to a reputable representative at your health food store are great ways to get the facts behind the products you take.

- **A history and trusted reputation.** Every product you buy comes from a company that has a history and a reputation. Be a wise consumer and don't be afraid to explore more about the company that you are considering as your supplement supplier. Always make sure the company that makes your supplements strictly adheres to Good Manufacturing Practices (cGMPs) and uses only the highest quality, scientifically validated ingredients. The FDA sets the cGMPs, and it's important any product you use should meet or exceed the requirements. Find out if the company you are considering does testing for strength, identity, purity, and composition. Once you have those answers, you'll know if it's a company you can trust.

- **Build a relationship with your local health food store.** The people who work there have a wealth of knowledge to share with you and are willing to take the time to talk about the specific health needs in your life. Most health food store owners and employees I have met across the country are there because they care, they know the supplements they sell, and they want to see people realize greater health without the side effects of pharmaceuticals.

☙ **Don't believe everything you read on the internet!** A good example is people talking about turmeric, which is a great spice. But a quick sound bite or post will falsely lead people to think that putting some turmeric spice on your food will yield the same results as published studies showing how curcumin, a compound in turmeric, delivered in a highly absorbable form can save lives. When you are putting something in your body, understand what it is, where it's from, how it was studied, how it works—including how it's getting to something as important as your cell—and what you should expect as an outcome. And the old adage still rings true; you get what you pay for. If something is much cheaper than comparable items, beware!

All the great herbs and botanicals in this book can make a difference when you begin with Vitamin YOU! I pray that each wonder of nature you choose will be used to lead you to a life filled with realized dreams, great joy, and vibrant health. You deserve nothing less.

In good health,
Terry Lemerond

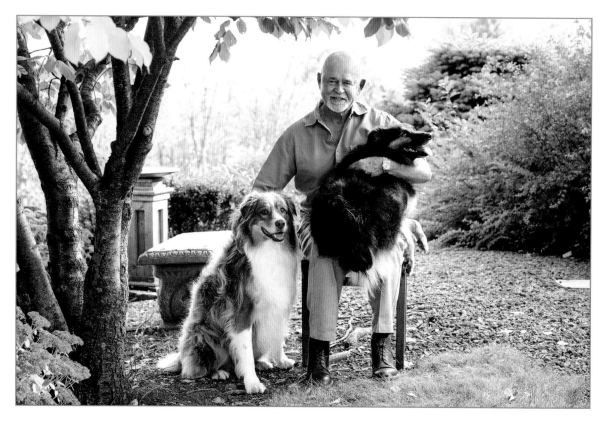

References

AMLA/INDIAN GOOSEBERRY

Antony B, Benny M, Kaimal TNB. A Pilot clinical study to evaluate the effect of *Emblica officinalis* extract (Amlamax™) on markers of systemic inflammation and dyslipidemia. *Indian Journal of Clinical Biochemistry*. 2008. 23.4, 378–381.

Baliga MS, Dsouza JJ. Amla (*Emblica officinalis* Gaertn), a wonder berry in the treatment and prevention of cancer. *Eur J Cancer Prev.* 2011 May;20(3):225–39.

ANDROGRAPHIS

Cáceres DD, Hancke JL, Burgos RA, Sandberg F, Wikman GK. Use of visual analogue scale measurements (VAS) to assess the effectiveness of standardized *Andrographis paniculata* extract SHA-10 in reducing the symptoms of common cold. A randomized double blind-placebo study. *Phytomedicine.* 1999 Oct;6(4):217–23.

Chandrasekaran CV, Thiyagarajan P, Sundarajan K, et al. Evaluation of the genotoxic potential and acute oral toxicity of standardized extract of *Andrographis paniculata* (KalmCold). *Food Chem Toxicol.* 2009;47(8):1892–902.

Coon JT, Ernst E. *Andrographis paniculata* in the treatment of upper respiratory tract infections: a systematic review of safety and efficacy. *Planta Med.* 2004;70(4):293–8.

Hossain MS, Urbi Z, Sule A, Hafizur Rahman KM. *Andrographis paniculata* (Burm. f.) Wall. ex Nees: a review of ethnobotany,

phytochemistry, and pharmacology. *Scientific World Journal.* 2014;2014:274905.

Ko HC, Wei BL, Chiou WF. The effect of medicinal plants used in Chinese folk medicine on RANTES secretion by virus-infected human epithelial cells. *J Ethnopharmacol.* 2006;107(2):205–10.

Lin TP, Chen SY, Duh PD, Chang LK, Liu YN. Inhibition of the epstein-barr virus lytic cycle by andrographolide. *Biol Pharm Bull.* 2008;31(11):2018–23.

Saxena RC, Singh R, Kumar P, Yadav SC, Negi MP, Saxena VS, Joshua AJ, Vijayabalaji V, Goudar KS, Venkateshwarlu K, Amit A. A randomized double blind placebo controlled clinical evaluation of extract of *Andrographis paniculata* (KalmCold) in patients with uncomplicated upper respiratory tract infection. *Phytomedicine.* 2010 Mar;17(3–4):178–85.

ANGELICA ARCHANGELICA

"Conditions Overview," from National Association for Continence. Available at: www.nafc.org/conditions-2/. Accessed: September 23, 2016.

"Overactive Bladder," from National Association for Continence. Available at: www.nafc.org/overactive-bladder. Accessed: September 23, 2016.

Cai X, Campbell N, Khan B, Callahan C, Boustani M. Long-term anticholinergic use and the aging brain. *Alzheimers Dement.* 2012 Nov 22.

Nitti VW. The Prevalence of Urinary Incontinence. *Reviews in Urology.* 2001;3(Suppl 1):S2–S6.

Sigurdsson S, Geirsson G, Gudmundsdottir H, Egilsdottir PB, Gudbjarnason S. A parallel, randomized, double-blind, placebo-controlled study to investigate the effect of a proprietary *Angelica archangelica* extract on nocturia in men. *Scand J Urol.* 2013 Feb;47(1):26–32.

Sigurdsson S, Gudbjarnason S. Inhibition of acetylcholinesterase by extracts and constituents from *Angelica archangelica* and *Geranium sylvaticum. Z Naturforsch C.* 2007 Sep-Oct,62(9–10):689–93.

Sigurdsson S, Ogmundsdottir HM, Gudbjarnason S. Antiproliferative effect of *Angelica archangelica* fruits. *Z Naturforsch C.* 2004 Jul-Aug;59(7–8):523–7.

Sigurdsson S, Ogmundsdottir HM, Gudbjarnason S. The cytotoxic effect of two chemotypes of essential oils from the fruits of *Angelica archangelica* L. *Anticancer Res.* 2005 May-Jun;25(3B):1877–80.

Sigurdsson S, Ogmundsdottir HM, Hallgrimsson J, Gudbjarnason S. Antitumour activity of *Angelica archangelica* leaf extract. *In Vivo.* 2005 Jan-Feb;19(1):191–4.

ASHWAGANDHA

Aalinkeel R, Hu Z, Nair BB, Sykes DE, Reynolds JL, Mahajan SD, Schwartz SA. Genomic Analysis Highlights the Role of the JAK-STAT Signaling in the Anti-proliferative Effects of Dietary Flavonoid—'Ashwagandha' in Prostate Cancer Cells. *Evid Based Complement Alternat Med.* 2010 Jun;7(2):177–187.

Alfaifi MY, Saleh KA, El-Boushnak MA, Elbehairi SE, Alshehri MA, Shati AA. Antiproliferative Activity of the Methanolic Extract of *Withania Somnifera* Leaves from Faifa Mountains, Southwest Saudi Arabia, against Several Human Cancer Cell Lines. *Asian Pac J Cancer Prev.* 2016;17(5):2723–2726.

Biswal BM, Sulaiman SA, Ismail HC, Zakaria H, Musa KI. Effect of *Withania somnifera* (Ashwagandha) on the development of chemotherapy-induced fatigue and quality of life in breast cancer patients. *Integr Cancer Ther.* 2013 Jul;12(4):312–322.

Choudhary D, Bhattacharyya S, Joshi K. Body Weight Management in Adults Under Chronic Stress Through Treatment With Ashwagandha Root Extract: A Double-Blind, Randomized, Placebo-Controlled Trial. *J Evid Based Complementary Altern Med.* 2016 Apr 6. Dar NJ, Hamid A, Ahmad M. Pharmacologic overview of *Withania somnifera*, the Indian Ginseng. *Cell Mol Life Sci.* 2015 Dec;72(23):4445–4460.

Gao R, Shah N, Lee JS, Katiyar SP, Li L, Oh E, Sundar D, Yun CO, Wadhwa R, Kaul SC. Withanone-rich combination of Ashwagandha withanolides restricts metastasis and angiogenesis through hnRNP-K. *Mol Cancer Ther.* 2014 Dec;13(12):2930–2940.

Halder B, Singh S, Thakur SS. *Withania somnifera* Root Extract Has Potent Cytotoxic Effect Against Human Malignant Melanoma Cells. *PLoS One.* 2015 Sep 3;10(9):e0137498.

Lee HE, Shin JA, Jeong JH, Jeon JG, Lee MH, Cho Sd. Anticancer activity of Ashwagandha against human head and neck cancer cell lines. *J Oral Pathol Med.* 2016 Mar;45(3):193–201.

McKenna MK, Gachuki BW, Alhakeem SS, Oben KN, Rangnekar VM, Gupta RC, Bondada S. Anti-cancer activity of withaferin A in B-cell lymphoma. *Cancer Biol Ther.* 2015;16(7):1088–1098.

Raguraman VR, Subramaniam JR. *Withania somnifera* Root Extract Enhances Telomerase Activity in the Human HeLa Cell Line. *Advances in Bioscience and Biotechnology.* 2016; 7:199–204.

Wankhede S, Langade D, Joshi K, Sinha SR, Bhattacharyya S. Examining the effect of *Withania somnifera* supplementation on muscle strength and recovery: a randomized controlled trial. *J Int Soc Sports Nutri.* 2015 Nov 25;12:43.

Widodo N, Takagi Y, Shrestha BG, Ishii T, Kaul SC, Wadhwa R. Selective killing of cancer cells by leaf extract of Ashwagandha: components, activity and pathway analyses. *Cancer Lett.* 2008 Apr;262(1):37–47.

ASTAXANTHIN

"Well-Known Antioxidants and Newcomers in Sport Nutrition: Coenzyme Q10, Quercetin, Resveratrol, Pterostilbene, Pycnogenol and Astaxanthin." Authors Belviranli M, Okudan N. Editors In: Lamprecht M, editor. *Antioxidants in Sport Nutrition.* Boca Raton (FL): CRC Press/Taylor & Francis; 2015. Chapter 5.

Aoi W, Naito Y, Takanami Y, et al. Astaxanthin improves muscle lipid metabolism in exercise via inhibitory effect of oxidative CPT I modification. *Biochem Biophys Res Commun.* 2008 Feb 22;366(4):892–7.

Aoi W, Naito Y, Takanami Y, Ishii T, Kawai Y, Akagiri S, Kato Y, Osawa T, Yoshikawa T. Astaxanthin improves muscle lipid metabolism in exercise via inhibitory effect of oxidative CPT I modification. *Biochem Biophys Res Commun.* 2008 Feb 22;366(4):892–7.

beCort A, Ozturk N, Akpinar D, *et al.* Suppressive effect of astaxanthin on retinal injury induced by elevated intraocular pressure. *Regul Toxicol Pharmacol.* 2010 Oct;58(1):121–30.

Choi HD, Kim JH, Chang MJ, Kyu-Youn Y, Shin WG. Effects of astaxanthin on oxidative stress in overweight and obese adults. *Phytother Res.* 2011 Dec;25(12):1813–8.

Choi HD, Youn YK, Shin WG. Positive effects of astaxanthin on lipid profiles and oxidative stress in overweight subjects. *Plant Foods Hum Nutr.* 2011 Nov;66(4):363–9.

Djordjevic B, Baralic I, Kotur-Stevuljevic J, *et al.* Effect of astaxanthin supplementation on muscle damage and oxidative stress markers in elite young soccer players. *J Sports Med Phys Fitness.* 2012 Aug;52(4):382–92.

Earnest CP, Lupo M, White KM, Church TS. Effect of astaxanthin on cycling time trial performance. *Int J Sports Med.* 2011 Nov;32(11):882–8.

Goto S, Kogure K, Abe K, et al. Efficient radical trapping at the surface and inside the phospholipid membrane is responsible for highly potent antiperoxidative activity of the carotenoid astaxanthin. *Biochim. Biophys. Acta.* 2001;1512:251–258.

Huang JY, Yeh PT, Hou YC. A randomized, double-blind, placebo-controlled study of oral antioxidant supplement therapy in patients with dry eye syndrome. *Clin Ophthalmol.* 2016 May 9;10:813–20.

Hussein G, Sankawa U, Goto H, Matsumoto K, Watanabe H. Astaxanthin, a carotenoid with potential in human health and nutrition. *J Nat Prod.* 2006;69(3):443–9.

Ikeuchi M, Koyama T, Takahashi J, Yazawa K. Effects of astaxanthin supplementation on exercise-induced fatigue in mice. *Biol Pharm Bull.* 2006 Oct;29(10):2106–10.

Karppi J, Rissanen TH, Nyyssönen K, et al. Effects of astaxanthin supplementation on lipid peroxidation. *Int J Vitam Nutr Res.* 2007 Jan;77(1):3–11.

Katagiri M, Satoh A, Tsuji S, Shirasawa T. Effects of astaxanthin-rich Haematococcus pluvialis extract on cognitive function: a randomised, double-blind, placebo-controlled study. *J Clin Biochem Nutr.* 2012 Sep;51(2):102–7.

Kidd P. Astaxanthin, cell membrane nutrient with diverse clinical benefits and anti-aging potential. *Altern Med Rev.* 2011 Dec;16(4):355–64.

Kishimoto Y, Yoshida H, Kondo K. Potential Anti-Atherosclerotic Properties of Astaxanthin. *Mar Drugs*. 2016 Feb 5;14(2). pii: E35.

Kishimoto Y, Yoshida H, Kondo K. Potential Anti-Atherosclerotic Properties of Astaxanthin. *Mar Drugs*. 2016 Feb 5;14(2). pii: E35.

Liu PH, Aoi W, Takami M, et al. The astaxanthin-induced improvement in lipid metabolism during exercise is mediated by a PGC-1[alpha] increase in skeletal muscle. *J Clin Biochem Nutr*. 2014 Mar;54(2):86–9.

Nagaki Y, Hayasaka S, Yamada T, Hayasaka Y, Sanada M, Uonomi T. Effects of astaxanthin on accommodation, critical flicker fusions, and pattern evoked potential in visual display terminal workers. *J. Trad. Med.*, 19(5):170–173, 2002.

Nakajima Y, Inokuchi Y, Shimazawa M, et al. Astaxanthin, a dietary carotenoid, protects retinal cells against oxidative stress in-vitro and in mice in-vivo. *J Pharm Pharmacol*. 2008;60(10):1365–74.

Park JS, Chyun JH, Kim YK, Line LL, Chew BP. Astaxanthin decreased oxidative stress and inflammation and enhanced immune response in humans. *Nutr Metab (Lond)*. 2010 Mar 5;7:18.

Yoshida H, Yanai H, Ito K, et al. Administration of natural astaxanthin increases serum HDL-cholesterol and adiponectin in subjects with mild hyperlipidemia. *Atherosclerosis*. 2010 Apr;209(2):520–3.

Yuan JP, Peng J, Yin K, Wang JH. Potential health-promoting effects of astaxanthin: a high-value carotenoid mostly from microalgae. *Mol Nutr Food Res*. 2011 Jan;55(1):150–65.

BLACK COHOSH

Schellenberg R, Saller R, Hess L, et al. Dependent Effects of the *Cimicifuga racemosa* Extract Ze 450 in the Treatment of Climacteric Complaints: A Randomized, Placebo-Controlled Study. *Evid Based Complement Alternat Med*. 2012; 2012:260301.

Wuttke W, Jarry H, Haunschild J, et al. The non-estrogenic alternative for the treatment of climacteric complaints: Black cohosh (*Cimicifuga or Actaea racemosa*). *J Steroid Biochem Mol Biol*. 2014 Jan;139:302–10.

BOSWELLIA FRANKINCENSE

Antony B, Kizhakedath R, Benny M, Kuruvilla BT. Clinical Evaluation of a herbal product (Rhulief™) in the management of knee osteoarthritis. Abstract 316. *Osteoarthritis Cartilage*. 2011;19(S1):S145–S146.

Catanzaro, Daniela, et al. *Boswellia serrata* preserves intestinal epithelial barrier from oxidative and inflammatory damage. *PloS one*. 2015; 10.5.

Gerhardt, H., et al. Therapy of active Crohn disease with *Boswellia serrata* extract H 15. *Zeitschrift fur Gastroenterologie*. 2001;39.1:11–17.

Goel, A. Boswellia extracts induce DNA methylation changes in colon cancer cells. Poster presentation, International Meeting of American Gastroenterological Association, Chicago, IL. 2011.

Gupta I, Gupta V, Parihar A, et al. Effects of *Boswellia serrata* gum resin in patients with bronchial asthma: results of a double-blind, placebo-controlled, 6-week clinical study. *Eur J Med Res*. 1998 Nov 17;3(11):511–4

Pungle P, Banavalikar M, Suthar A, Biyani M, Mengi S. Immunomodulatory activity of boswellic acids of *Boswellia serrata* Roxb. *Indian J Exp Biol*. 2003 Dec;41(12):1460–2.

BUTCHER'S BROOM

Aguilar Peralta GR, Arévalo Gardoqui J, Llamas Macías FJ, Navarro Ceja VH, Mendoza Cisneros SA, Martínez Macías CG. Clinical and capillaroscopic evaluation in the treatment of chronic venous insufficiency with *Ruscus aculeatus*, hesperidin methylchalcone and ascorbic acid in venous insufficiency treatment of ambulatory patients. *Int Angiol.* 2007 Dec;26(4):378–84.

Guex JJ, Avril L, Enrici E, Enriquez E, Lis C, Taïeb C. Quality of life improvement in Latin American patients suffering from chronic venous disorder using a combination of *Ruscus aculeatus* and hesperidin methyl-chalcone and ascorbic acid (quality study). *Int Angiol.* 2010 Dec;29(6):525–32.

Guex JJ, Enrici E, Boussetta S, Avril L, Lis C, Taieb C. Correlations between ankle circumference, symptoms, and quality of life demonstrate the clinical relevance of minimal leg swelling reduction: results of a study in 1,036 Argentinean patients. *Dermatol Surg.* 2008 Dec;34(12):1666–75.

Huang YL, Kou JP, Ma L, Song JX, Yu BY. Possible mechanism of the anti-inflammatory activity of ruscogenin: role of intercellular adhesion molecule-1 and nuclear factor-kappaB. *J Pharmacol Sci.* 2008 Oct;108(2):198–205.

Redman DA. *Ruscus aculeatus* (butcher's broom) as a potential treatment for orthostatic hypotension, with a case report. *J Altern Complement Med.* 2000 Dec;6(6):539–49.

Ruscus aculeatus (butcher's broom). Monograph. *Altern Med Rev.* 2001 Dec;6(6):608–12.

Vanscheidt W, Jost V, Wolna P, Lücker PW, Müller A, Theurer C, Patz B, Grützner KI. Efficacy and safety of a Butcher's broom preparation (*Ruscus aculeatus L.* extract) compared to placebo in patients suffering from chronic venous insufficiency. *Arzneimittelforschung.* 2002;52(4):243–50.

CAT'S CLAW

Aguilar JL, Rojas P, Marcelo A, et al. Anti-inflammatory activity of two different extracts of *Uncaria tomentosa* (Rubiaceae). *Journal of Ethnopharmacology* 81, no. 2:2002. 271–276.

alkaloids from *Uncaria tomentosa* (cat's claw): Chemotype relevance. J

Apr–May:35–6. Spanish.

Dreifuss AA, Bastos-Pereira AL, Avila TV, et al. Antitumoral and antioxidant effects of a hydroalcoholic extract of cat's claw (Uncaria tomentosa) (Willd. Ex Roem. & Schult) in an in vivo carcinosarcoma model. *J Ethnopharmacol.* 2010 Jul 6;130(1):127–33.

Ethnopharmacol. 2016 Aug 2;189:90–8.

Jalloh MA, Gregory PJ, Hein D, et al. Dietary supplement interactions with antiretrovirals: a systematic review. *Int J STDAIDS.* 2016 Sep 21.

Kaiser S, Carvalho ÂR, Pittol V, et al. Genotoxicity and cytotoxicity of oxindole

Lamm S, Sheng Y, Pero, RW. Persistent response to pneumococcal vaccine in individuals supplemented with a novel water soluble extract of *Uncaria tomentosa*, C-Med-100®. *Phytomedicine* 2001. 8.4: 267–274.

Muhammad I, Dunbar C, Khan RA, et al. Investigation of Una De Gato I. 7-Deoxyloganic acid and 15 N NMR spectroscopic studies on pentacyclic oxindole alkaloids from *Uncaria tomentosa. Phytochemistry* 57, no. 5: 2001. 781–785.

Mur E, Hartig F, Eibl G, Schirmer M. Randomized double blind trial of an extract from the pentacyclic alkaloid-chemotype of uncaria tomentosa for the treatment of rheumatoid arthritis. *J Rheumatol.* 2002 Apr;29(4):678–81.

Sandoval, Manuel, Randi M. et al. Cat's claw inhibits TNF[alpha] production and scavenges free radicals: role in cytoprotection. *Free Radical Biology and Medicine* 29, no. 1: 2000. 71–78.

Sheng Y, Li L, Holmgren K, et al. DNA repair enhancement of aqueous extracts of *Uncaria tomentosa* in a human volunteer study. *Phytomedicine* 8, no. 4: 2001. 275–282.

Sheng Y, Pero RW, Wagner H. Treatment of chemotherapy-induced leukopenia in a rat model with aqueous extract from *Uncaria tomentosa*. *Phytomedicine* 2000. 7.2: 137–143.

Steinberg PN. [Cat's Claw: an herb from the Peruvian Amazon]. *Sidahora*. 1995

Stuppner H, Sturm S, and Konwalinka G. HPLC analysis of the main oxindole alkaloids from *Uncaria tomentosa*. *Chromatographia* 1992.34.11–12: 597–600.

CHASTEBERRY

Ambrosini A, Di Lorenzo C, Coppola G, et al. Use of *Vitex agnus-castus* in migrainous women with premenstrual syndrome: an open-label clinical observation. *Acta Neurol Belg.* 2013 Mar;113(1):25–9.

Ghanbari Z, Haghollahi F, Shariat M, et al. Effects of calcium supplement therapy in women with premenstrual syndrome. *Taiwan J Obstet Gynecol.* 2009 Jun;48(2):124–129.

Schellenberg R, Zimmermann C, Drewe J, et al. Dose-dependent efficacy of the *Vitex agnus castus* extract Ze 440 in patients suffering from premenstrual syndrome. *Phytomedicine.* 2012 Nov 15;19(14):1325–31.

Schellenberg R. Treatment for the premenstrual syndrome with agnus castus fruit extract: prospective, randomised, placebo controlled study. *BMJ.* 2001 January 20; 322(7279): 134–137.

Sohrabi N, Kashanian M, Ghafoori SS, et al. Evaluation of the effect of omega-3 fatty acids in the treatment of premenstrual syndrome: "a pilot trial." *Complement Ther Med.* 2013 Jun;21(3):141–6.

Zamani M, Neghab N, Torabian S. Therapeutic effect of *Vitex agnus castus* in patients with premenstrual syndrome. *Acta Med Iran.* 2012;50(2):101–6.

CHERRY FRUIT

Bell PG, Gaze DC, Davison GW, et al. Montmorency tart cherry (*Prunus cerasus L.*) concentrate lowers uric acid, independent of plasma cyanidin-3-O-glucosiderutinoside. *Journal of Functional Foods.* 2014; 11: 82–90

Howatson G, Bell PG, Tallent J, et al. Effect of tart cherry juice (*Prunus cerasus*) on melatonin levels and enhanced sleep quality." *European Journal of Nutrition* 51, no. 8: 201

Howatson G, McHugh MP, Hill JA, et al. Influence of tart cherry juice on indices of recovery following marathon running. *Scand. J. Med. Sci. Sports.* 2010;20:843–852.

Kuehl K, Perrier E, Elliot D, et al. Efficacy of tart cherry juice in reducing muscle pain during running: A randomized controlled trial. *J. Int. Soc. Sports Nutr.* 2010;7:17.

Zhang Y, Neogi T, Chen,C, et al. (2012), Cherry consumption and decreased risk of recurrent gout attacks. *Arthritis & Rheumatism.* 64: 4004–4011.

COMFREY

Barna M, Kucera A, Hladíkova M, Kucera M. Randomized double-blind study: wound-healing effects of a Symphytum herb extract cream (*Symphytum x uplandicum* Nyman) in children. *Arzneimittelforschung.* 2012 Jun;62(6):285–9.

Durso GR, Luttrell A, Way BM. Over-the-Counter Relief from Pains and Pleasures Alike: Acetaminophen Blunts Evaluation Sensitivity to Both Negative and Positive Stimuli. *Psychol Sci.*2015 Jun;26(6):750–758.

Earnest DL. NSAID-induced gastric injury: its pathogenesis and management. *Semin Arthritis Rheum*. 1990 Feb;19(4 Suppl 2):6–10.

Grünwald J, Bitterlich N, Nauert C, Schmidt, M. Application and safety of comfrey cream (*Symphyti herba*) in paediatric treatment of acute blunt traumata (Anwendung und Verträglichkeit von Beinwellcreme (*Symphyti herba*) bei Kindern mit akuten stumpfen Traumen). Anwendung und Verträglichkeit von Beinwellcreme (*Symphyti herba*) bei Kindern mit akuten stumpfen Traumen. *Z Phytother*. 2010;31:61–65.

Hess H. Effect of a Symphytum ointment with sports injuries of the knee joint. *Dtsch Z Sportmed* [*German J Sports Med*]. 1991;42(4):156–162.

Jones RH, Tait CL. Gastrointestinal side-effects of NSAIDs in the community. *Br J Clin Pract*. 1995 Mar-Apr;49(2):67–70.

Schmidt M. Topic: High-performance cultivar 'Harras' as a contribution to quality, efficacy and safety of comfrey (Symphytum x uplandicum Nyman). [Thema: High-performance cultivar 'Harras' as a contribution to quality, efficacy and safety of comfrey (*Symphytum x uplandicum Nyman*] *Z Arznei-Gewurzpfla*. 2008;13(4):182–183. [German].

Süleyman H, Demircan B, Karagöz Y. Anti-inflammatory and side effects of cyclo-oxygenase inhibitors. *Pharmacol Rep*. 2007 May-Jun;59(3):247–258.

Uebelhack R, Shaudt M, Schmidt M. Beinwell-Herba-Extrakt-Crème zur Schmerzlinderung bei traininginduziertem Muskelkater—eine randomisierte placebokontrollierte Studie. *J Pharmakol Therap*. 2014;23(1):3.

Weir MR. Renal effects of nonselective NSAIDs and coxibs. *Cleve Clin J Med*. 2002;69 Suppl 1:SI53–58.

COQ10

Deichmann R, Lavie C, Andrews S. Coenzyme q10 and statin-induced mitochondrial dysfunction. *Ochsner J*. 2010 Spring;10(1):16–21.

Del Pozo-Cruz J, Rodríguez-Bies E, Navas-Enamorado I, Del Pozo-Cruz B, Navas P, López-Lluch G.Relationship between functional capacity and body mass index with plasma coenzyme Q10 and oxidative damage in community-dwelling elderly-people. *Exp Gerontol*. 2014 Apr;52:46–54.

Garrido-Maraver J, Cordero MD, Oropesa-Ávila M, *et al*. Coenzyme q10 therapy. *Mol Syndromol*. 2014 Jul;5(3–4):187–197.

Hodgson JM, Watts GF, Playford DA, et al. Coenzyme Q(10) improves blood pressure and glycaemic control: a controlled trial in subjects with type 2 diabetes. *Eur J Clin Nutr*. 2002;56:1137–1142.

Litarru G. P., Tiano L. Bioenergetic and antioxidant properties of coenzyme Q10: recent developments. *Mol Biotechnol*. 2007;37:31–37.

Markley HG. CoEnzyme Q10 and riboflavin: the mitochondrial connection. *Headache*. 2012 Oct;52 Suppl 2:81–87.

Mortensen SA, Rosenfeldt F, Kumar A, *et al*. The Effect of Coenzyme Q10 on Morbidity and Mortality in Chronic Heart Failure: Results From Q-SYMBIO: A Randomized Double-Blind Trial. *JACC Heart Fail*. 2014 Dec;2(6):641–649

Muroyama A. An alternative medical approach for the neuroprotective therapy to slow the progression of Parkinson's disease. *Yakugaku Zasshi*. 2013;133(8):849–856.

Norata GD, Tibolla G, Catapano AL. Statins and skeletal muscles toxicity: from clinical trials to everyday practice. *Pharmacol Res*. 2014 Oct;88:107–113

Parkinson's Study Group. A randomized clinical trial of high-dosage coenzyme Q10 in early Parkinson disease: no evidence of benefit. *JAMA Neurol.* 2014 May;71(5):543–552.

Pourmoghaddas M, Rabbani M, Shahabi J, Garakyaraghi M, Khanjani R, Hedayat P. Combination of atorvastatin/coenzyme Q10 as adjunctive treatment in congestive heart failure: A double-blind randomized placebo-controlled clinical trial. *ARYA Atheroscler.* 2014 Jan;10(1):1–5.

Rosenfeldt FL, Haas SJ, Krum H, *et al. Coenzyme Q10 in the treatment of hypertension: a meta-analysis of the clinical trials.* J Hum Hypertens. *2007 Apr;21(4):297–306.*

Shults CW, Oakes D, Kieburtz K, et al. *Effects of coenzyme Q10 in early Parkinson disease: evidence of slowing of the functional decline.* Arch Neurol. *2002 Oct;59(10):1541–550.*

Wyman M, Leonard M, Morledge T. Coenzyme Q10: a therapy for hypertension and statin-induced myalgia? Cleve Clin J Med. *2010 Jul;77(7):435–442.*

Yorns WR Jr, Hardison HH. Mitochondrial dysfunction in migraine. Semin Pediatr Neurol. *2013 Sep;20(3):188–193.*

CURCUMIN

Aggarwal BB, Kumar A, Bharti AC. Anticancer potential of curcumin: preclinical and clinical studies. *Anticancer Res.* 2003 Jan-Feb;23(1A):363–98.

Aggarwal BB, Sundaram C, Malani N, Ichikawa H. Curcumin: the Indian solid gold. *Adv Exp Med Biol.* 2007;595:1–75.

Aggarwal BB, Yuan W, Li S, Gupta SC. Curcumin-free turmeric exhibits anti-inflammatory and anticancer activities: Identification of novel components of turmeric. *Mol Nutr Food Res.* 2013 Sep;57(9):1529–42.

Antony B, Kizhakedath R, Benny M, Kuruvilla BT. Clinical Evaluation of a herbal product (Rhulief™) in the management of knee osteoarthritis. Abstract 316. *Osteoarthritis Cartilage.* 2011;19(S1):S145-S146.

Antony B, Merina B, Iyer VS, et al. A Pilot Cross-Over Study to Evaluate Human Oral Bioavailability of BCM-95CG (Biocurcumax), A Novel Bioenhanced Preparation of Curcumin. *Indian J Pharm Sci.* 2008; 70(4):445–449.

Benny M, Antony B. Bioavailability of BioCurcumax™ (BCM-095™). *Spice India.* September, 2006 :11–15.

Bereswill S, Muñoz M, Fischer A, et al. Anti-inflammatory effects of resveratrol, curcumin and simvastatin in acute small intestinal inflammation. *PLoS One.* 2010;5(12):e15099.

Buhrmann C, Kraehe P, Lueders C, Shayan P, Goel A, et al. Curcumin Suppresses Crosstalk between Colon Cancer Stem Cells and Stromal Fibroblasts in the Tumor Microenvironment: Potential Role of EMT. *PLoS ONE.* 2014;9(9): e107514

Bundy R, Walker AF, Middleton RW, Booth J. Turmeric extract may improve irritable bowel syndrome symptomology in otherwise healthy adults: a pilot study. *J Altern Complement Med.* 2004 Dec;10(6):1015–8.

Chandran B, Goel A. A Randomized, Pilot Study to Assess the Efficacy and Safety of Curcumin in Patients with Active Rheumatoid Arthritis. *Phytother Res.* March 9, 2012 doi: 10.1002/ptr.4639.

Cheng AL, Hsu CH, Lin JK, Hsu MM, et al. Phase I clinical trial of curcumin, a chemopreventive agent, in patients with high-risk or pre-malignant lesions. *Anticancer Res.* 2001;21:2895–900.

Deepa Das A, Balan A, Sreelatha KT. Comparative study of the efficacy of curcumin and turmeric as chemopreventive agents in oral submucous fibrosis: a clinical and histopathological evaluation. *JIAOMR;* April-June 2010;22(2):88–92.

Drobnic F, Riera J, Appendino G, Togni S, Franceschi F, Valle X, Pons A, Tur J. Reduction of delayed onset muscle soreness by a novel curcumin delivery system (Meriva®): a randomised, placebo-controlled trial. *J Int Soc Sports Nutr*. 2014 Jun 18;11:31.

Ejaz A, Wu D, Kwan P, Meydani M. Curcumin inhibits adipogenesis in 3T3-L1 adipocytes and angiogenesis and obesity in C57/BL mice. *J Nutr*. 2009 May;139(5):919–25.

El-Moselhy MA, Taye A, Sharkawi SS, El-Sisi SF, Ahmed AF. The antihyperglycemic effect of curcumin in high fat diet fed rats. Role of TNF-[alpha] and free fatty acids. *Food Chem Toxicol*. 2011;49(5):1129–40.

Garcia-Alloza M. Curcumin labels amyloid pathology in vivo, disrupts existing plaques, and partially restores distorted neurites in an Alzheimer mouse model. *J Neurochem*. 2007;102:1095–1104.

Gaziano JM, Hennekens CH, O'Donnell CJ, Breslow JL, Buring JE. Fasting triglycerides, high-density lipoprotein, and risk of myocardial infarction. *Circulation*. 1997;96(8):2520–5.

Goel A, Aggarwal BB. Curcumin, the golden spice from Indian saffron, is a chemosensitizer and radiosensitizer for tumors and chemoprotector and radioprotector for normal organs. *Nutr Cancer*. 2010;62(7):919–30.

Goel A, Jhurani S, Aggarwal BB. Multi-targeted therapy by curcumin: how spicy is it? *Mol Nutr Food Res*. 2008;52(9):1010–30.

Gupta SC, Patchva S, Koh W, Aggarwal BB. Discovery of Curcumin, a Component of the Golden Spice, and Its Miraculous Biological Activities. *Clin Exp Pharmacol Physiol*. 2011.

Gupta SK, Kumar B, Nag TC, et al. Curcumin prevents experimental diabetic retinopathy in rats through its hypoglycemic, antioxidant, and anti-inflammatory mechanisms. *J Ocul Pharmacol Ther*. 2011; 27(2):123–30

Hejazi J, Rastmanesh R, Taleban F, Molana S, and Ehtejab G. A Pilot Clinical Trial of Radioprotective Effects of Curcumin Supplementation in Patients with Prostate Cancer. *J Cancer Sci Ther*. 2013, 5.10.

Henrotin Y, Clutterbuck AL, Allaway D, et al. Biological actions of curcumin on articular chondrocytes. *Osteoarthritis Cartilage*. 2010;18(2):141–9.

Holt PR, Katz S, Kirshoff R. Curcumin therapy in inflammatory bowel disease: a pilot study. *Dig Dis Sci*. 2005;50(11):2191–3.

Huang Z, Zhong XM, Li ZY, Feng CR, Pan AJ, Mao QQ. Curcumin reverses corticosterone-induced depressive-like behavior and decrease in brain BDNF levels in rats. *Neurosci Lett*. 2011;493(3):145–8.

Hucklenbroich J, Klein R, Neumaier B, Graf R, Fink GR, Schroeter M, Rueger MA. Aromatic-turmerone induces neural stem cell proliferation in vitro and in vivo. *Stem Cell Res Ther*. 2014 Sep 26;5(4):100.

Jagetia GC, Rajanikant GK. Effect of curcumin on radiation-impaired healing of excisional wounds in mice. *J Wound Care*. 2004 Mar;13(3):107–9.

Johnson JJ, Mukhtar H. Curcumin for chemoprevention of colon cancer. *Cancer Lett*. 2007;255(2):170–81.

Kulkarni SK, Dhir A. An overview of curcumin in neurological disorders. *Indian J Pharm Sci*. 2010;72(2):149–54.

Liju VB, Jeena K, Kuttan R. An evaluation of antioxidant, anti-inflammatory, and antinociceptive activities of essential oil from Curcuma longa. L. *Indian J Pharmacol*. 2011 Sep;43(5):526–31.

Lopresti AL, Drummond PD. Efficacy of curcumin, and a saffron/curcumin combination for the treatment of major depression: A randomised, double-blind, placebo-controlled study. *J Affect Disord*. 2016 Oct 1;207:188–196.

Lopresti AL, Maes M, Maker GL, Hood S, Drummond PD. Curcumin and major depression: A randomized, double-blind, placebo-controlled trial investigating the potential of peripheral biomarkers to predict treatment response and antidepressant mechanisms of change. *European Neuropsychopharmacology.* 2014. Dec. 5.

Lopresti AL, Maes M, Maker GL, Hood S, Drummond PD. Curcumin for the treatment of major depression: A randomised, double-blind, placebo controlled study. *J Affect Disord.* 2014;167:368–375.

Martins R. Evaluation of the nutritional extract Bio-curcumin (BCM-95) to preserve cognitive functioning in a cohort of mild cognitively impaired (MCI) patients over 12 months. Edith Cowan University. Joondalup, Western Australia.

Meeran SM, Ahmed A, Tollefsbol TO. Epigenetic targets of bioactive dietary components for cancer prevention and therapy. *Clin Epigenetics.* 2010;1(3–4):101–116.

Murakami A, Furukawa I, Miyamoto S, Tanaka T, Ohigashi H. Curcumin combined with turmerones, essential oil components of turmeric, abolishes inflammation-associated mouse colon carcinogenesis. *Biofactors.* 2013 Mar-Apr;39(2):221–32.

Na LX, Zhang YL, Li Y, et al. Curcumin improves insulin resistance in skeletal muscle of rats. *Nutr Metab Cardiovasc Dis.* 2011 Jul;21(7):526–33.

Nicol LM, Rowlands DS, Fazakerly R, Kellett J. Curcumin supplementation likely attenuates delayed onset muscle soreness (DOMS). *Eur J Appl Physiol.* 2015 Aug;115(8):1769–77.

Orellana-Paucar AM, Afrikanova T, Thomas J, Aibuldinov YK, Dehaen W, de Witte PA, Esguerra CV. Insights from zebrafish and mouse models on the activity and safety of ar-turmerone as a potential drug candidate for the treatment of epilepsy. *PLoS One.* 2013 Dec 13;8(12):e81634.

Park SY, Jin ML, Kim YH, Kim Y, Lee SJ. Anti-inflammatory effects of aromatic-turmerone through blocking of NF-[kappa]B, JNK, and p38 MAPK signaling pathways in amyloid [beta]-stimulated microglia. *Int Immunopharmacol.* 2012 Sep;14(1):13–20.

Peeyush KT, Gireesh G, Jobin M, Paulose CS. Neuroprotective role of curcumin in the cerebellum of streptozotocin-induced diabetic rats. *Life Sci.* 2009;85(19–20):704–10.

Rajasekaran SA. Therapeutic potential of curcumin in gastrointestinal diseases. *World J Gastrointest Pathophysiol.* 2011;2(1):1–14.

Rungseesantivanon S, Thenchaisri N, Ruangvejvorachai P, Patumraj S. Curcumin supplementation could improve diabetes-induced endothelial dysfunction associated with decreased vascular superoxide production and PKC inhibition. *BMC Complement Altern Med.* 2010;10:57.

Sanmukhani J, Anovadiya A, Tripathi CB. Evaluation of Antidepressant Like Activity of Curcumin and its Combination with Fluoxetine and Imipramine: an Acute and Chronic Study. *Acta Pol Pharm.* 2011 Sep-Oct;68(5):769–75.

Sanmukhani J, Satodia V, Trivedi J, Patel T, Tiwari D, Panchal B, Goel A, Tripathi CB. Efficacy and safety of curcumin in major depressive disorder: a randomized controlled trial. *Phytother Res.* 2013;28(4):579–85.

Sciberras JN, Galloway SD, Fenech A, Grech G, Farrugia C, Duca D, Mifsud J. The effect of turmeric (Curcumin) supplementation on cytokine and inflammatory marker responses following 2 hours of endurance cycling. *J Int Soc Sports Nutr.* 2015 Jan 21;12(1):5.

Seo KI, Choi MS, Jung UJ, et al. Effect of curcumin supplementation on blood glucose, plasma insulin, and glucose homeostasis related enzyme activities in diabetic db/db mice. *Mol Nutr Food Res.* 2008; 52(9):995–1004.

Shakibaei M, Buhrmann C, Kraehe P, Shayan P, Lueders C and Goel A. Curcumin chemosensitizes 5-Fluorouracil resistant MMR-deficient human colon cancer cells in high density cultures. *PLoS ONE*. 2014:9(1).

Shehzad A, Wahid F, Lee YS. Curcumin in cancer chemoprevention: molecular targets, pharmacokinetics, bioavailability, and clinical trials. *Arch Pharm (Weinheim)*. 2010; 343(9):489–99.

Shin SK, HA TY, McGregor RA, Choi MS. Long-term curcumin administration protects against atherosclerosis via hepatic regulation of lipoprotein cholesterol metabolism. *Mol Nutr Food Res*. 2011 Nov 7.

Sidhu GS, Mani H, Gaddipati JP, Singh AK, et al. Curcumin enhances wound healing in streptozotocin induced diabetic rats and genetically diabetic mice. *Wound Repair Regen*. 1999 Sep-Oct;7(5):362–74.

Soni KB, Kuttan R. Effect of oral curcumin administration on serum peroxides and cholesterol levels in human volunteers. *Indian J Physiol Pharmacol*. 1992 Oct;36(4):273–5.

Thangapazham RL, Sharma A, Maheshwari RK. Beneficial role of curcumin in skin diseases. *Adv Exp Med Biol*. 2007;595:343–57.

Xu Y, Ku BS, Yao HY, et al. The effects of curcumin on depressive-like behaviors in mice. *Eur J Pharmacol*. 2005;518(1):40–6.

DEVIL'S CLAW

Brendler T, Gruenwald J, Ulbricht C, and Basch E. Devil's Claw (*Harpagophytum procumbens* DC) An Evidence-Based Systematic Review by the Natural Standard Research Collaboration. *Journal of Herbal Pharmacotherapy*. 2006 6(1), pp.89–126.

Chrubasik S, Mode, A, Black A, and Pollak S. A randomized double-blind pilot study comparing Doloteffin® and Vioxx® in the treatment of low back pain. *Rheumatology*. 2003 42(1), pp.141–148.

Georgiev MI, Ivanovska N, Alipieva K, Dimitrova P, Verpoorte R.. Harpagoside: from Kalahari Desert to pharmacy shelf. *Phytochemistry*.2013 92, pp.8–15.

Sanders M and Grundmann O. The use of glucosamine, devil's claw (*Harpagophytum procumbens*), and acupuncture as complementary and alternative treatments for osteoarthritis. *Altern Med Rev*. 2011 16(3), pp.228–238.

Warnock M, McBean D, Suter A, Tan J. and Whittaker, P. Effectiveness and safety of Devil's Claw tablets in patients with general rheumatic disorders. *Phytotherapy Research*. 2007 21(12), pp.1228–1233.

Wegener T, Lüpke NP. Treatment of patients with arthrosis of hip or knee with an aqueous extract of devil's claw (*Harpagophytum procumbens* DC.). *Phytotherapy Research*. 2003 17(10), pp.1165–1172.

D-RIBOSE

Omran H, Illien S, MacCarter D, St Cyr J, Lüderitz B. D-Ribose improves diastolic function and quality of life in congestive heart failure patients: a prospective feasibility study. *Eur J Heart Fail*. 2003 Oct;5(5):615–9.

Omran H, McCarter D, St Cyr J, Lüderitz B. D-ribose aids congestive heart failure patients. *Exp Clin Cardiol*. 2004 Summer;9(2):117–8.

Teitelbaum JE, Johnson C, St Cyr J. The use of D-ribose in chronic fatigue syndrome and fibromyalgia: a pilot study. *J Altern Complement Med*. 2006 Nov;12(9):857–62

ECHINACEA

Ardjomand-Woelkart K, Bauer R. Review and Assessment of Medicinal Safety Data of Orally

Used Echinacea Preparations. *Planta Med.* 2016 Jan;82(1-2):17–31.

Delorme D, Miller SC. Dietary consumption of Echinacea by mice afflicted with autoimmune (type I) diabetes: effect of consuming the herb on hemopoietic and immune cell dynamics. *Autoimmunity.* 2005 Sep;38(6):453–461.

Hájos N, Holderith N, Németh B, et al. The effects of an Echinacea preparation on synaptic transmission and the firing properties of CA1 pyramidal cells in the hippocampus. *Phytother Res.*2012 Mar;26(3):354–362.

Haller J, Freund TF, Pelczer KG, Füredi J, Krecsak L, Zámbori J. The anxiolytic potential and psychotropic side effects of an echinacea preparation in laboratory animals and healthy volunteers. *Phytother Res.* 2013 Jan;27(1):54–61.

Haller J, Hohmann J, Freund TF. The effect of Echinacea preparations in three laboratory tests of anxiety: comparison with chlordiazepoxide. *Phytother Res.* 2010 Nov;24(11):1605–13.

Jawad M, Schoop R, Suter A, Klein P, Eccles R. Safety and Efficacy Profile of Echinacea purpurea to Prevent Common Cold Episodes: A Randomized, Double-Blind, Placebo-Controlled Trial. *Evid Based Complement Alternat Med.* 2012;2012:841315.

Nahas R, Balla A. Complementary and alternative medicine for prevention and treatment of the common cold. *Can Fam Physician.* 2011 Jan;57(1):31–6.

Neri PG, Stagni E, Filippello M, Camillieri G, Giovannini A, Leggio GM, Drago F. Oral Echinacea purpurea extract in low-grade, steroid-dependent, autoimmune idiopathic uveitis: a pilot study. *J Ocul Pharmacol Ther.* 2006 Dec;22(6):431–436.

ELDERBERRY

Krawitz C, Mraheil MA, Stein M, et al. Inhibitory activity of a standardized elderberry liquid extract against clinically-relevant human respiratory bacterial pathogens and influenza A and B viruses. *BMC Complement Altern Med.* 2011 Feb 25;11:16.

Ozgen M, Scheerens JC, Reese RN, Miller RA. Total phenolic, anthocyanin contents and antioxidant capacity of selected elderberry (*Sambucus canadensis L.*) accessions. *Pharmacogn Mag.* 2010 Jul;6(23):198–203.

Roschek B Jr, Fink RC, McMichael MD, Li D, Alberte RS. Elderberry flavonoids bind to and prevent H1N1 infection in vitro. *Phytochemistry.* 2009 Jul;70(10):1255–61.

Roschek B Jr, Fink RC, McMichael MD, Li D, Alberte RS. Elderberry flavonoids bind to and prevent H1N1 infection in vitro. *Phytochemistry.* 2009 Jul;70(10):1255–61.

Tiralongo E, Wee SS, Lea RA. Elderberry Supplementation Reduces Cold Duration and Symptoms in Air-Travellers: A Randomized, Double-Blind Placebo-Controlled Clinical Trial. *Nutrients.* 2016 Mar 24;8(4):182.

Vlachojannis JE, Cameron M, Chrubasik S. A systematic review on the *sambuci fructus* effect and efficacy profiles. *Phytother Res.* 2010 Jan;24(1):1–8

ELEUTHERO

Asano K, Takahashi T, Miyashita M, et al. Effect of *Eleutheroccocus senticosus* Extract on Human Physical Working Capacity. *Planta Med.* 1986;52(3):175–177

Cicero AF, Derosa G, Brillante R, Bernardi R, Nascetti S, Gaddi A. Effects of Siberian ginseng (*Eleutherococcus senticosus* maxim.) on elderly quality of life: a randomized clinical trial. *Arch Gerontol Geriatr Suppl.* 2004;(9):69–73

Facchinetti F, Neri I, Tarabusi M. *Eleutherococcus senticosus* reduces cardiovascular response in healthy subjects: a randomized, placebo-controlled trial. *Stress Health.* 2002;18:11–17.

Hartz AJ, Bentler S, Noyes R, et al. Randomized controlled trial of Siberian ginseng for chronic fatigue. *Psychol Med.* 2004;34:51–61.

Huang LZ, Wei L, Zhao HF, Huang BK, Rahman K, Qin LP. The effect of Eleutheroside E on behavioral alterations in murine sleep deprivation stress model. *Eur J Pharmacol.* 2011 May 11;658(2–3):150–155.

Kimura Y, Sumiyoshi M. Effects of various *Eleutherococcus senticosus* cortex on swimming time, natural killer activity and corticosterone level in forced swimming stressed mice. *J Ethnopharmacol.* 2004;95(2–3):447–453.

Panossian A, Wikman G, Kaur P, Asea A. Adaptogens stimulate neuropeptide y and hsp72 expression and release in neuroglia cells. *Front Neurosci.* 2012 Feb 1;6:6.

Panossian A, Wikman G. Evidence-based efficacy of adaptogens in fatigue, and molecular mechanisms related to their stress-protective activity. *Curr Clin Pharmacol.* 2009 Sep;4(3):198–219.

EUCALYPTUS

Cermelli C, Fabio A, Fabio G, Quaglio P. Effect of eucalyptus essential oil on respiratory bacteria and viruses. *Curr Microbiol.* 2008;56(1):89–92.

Hong CZ, and Shellock FG. Effects of a Topically Applied Counterirritant (Eucalyptamint) on Cutaneous Blood Flow and on Skin and Muscle Temperatures: A Placebo-Controlled Study. *American Journal of Physical Medicine & Rehabilitation.* 1991. 70.1: 29–33.

Juergens U R, Dethlefsen U, Steinkamp G, et al. Anti-inflammatory activity of 1,8 cineole (eucalpytol) in bronchial asthma: a double blind, placebo controlled trial. *Respir Med.* 2003;97(3)250–256.

Mulyaningsih S. Antibacterial activity of essential oils from Eucalyptus and of selected components against multidrug-resistant bacterial pathogens. *Pharm Biol.* 2011;49(9):893–9.

Salari MH, Amine G, Shirazi MH, Hafezi R, Mohammadypour M. Antibacterial effects of *Eucalyptus globulus* leaf extract on pathogenic bacteria isolated from specimens of patients with respiratory tract disorders. *Clin Microbiol Infect.* 2006;12(2):194–6.

Silva J, Abebe W, Sousa SM, Duarte VG, Machado MI, Matos FJ. Analgesic and anti-inflammatory effects of essential oils of Eucalyptus. *J Ethnopharmacol.* 2003;89(2–3):277–83.

FIBER

Kaats GR, Michalek JE, Preuss HG. Evaluating efficacy of a chitosan product using a double-blinded, placebo-controlled protocol. *J Am Coll Nutr.* 2006 Oct;25(5):389–94.

Kerch G. The potential of chitosan and its derivatives in prevention and treatment of age-related diseases. *Mar Drugs.* 2015 Apr 13;13(4):2158–82.

Kim HJ, Ahn HY, Kwak JH, et al. The effects of chitosan oligosaccharide (GO2KA1) supplementation on glucose control in subjects with prediabetes. *Food Funct.* 2014 Oct;5(10):2662–9.

Lodhi G, Kim YS, Hwang JW, et al. Chitooligosaccharide and its derivatives: preparation and biological applications. *Biomed Res Int.* 2014;2014:654913.

Mendis E, Kim MM, Rajapakse N, Kim SK. An in vitro cellular analysis of the radical scavenging efficacy of chitooligosaccharides. *Life Sci.* 2007 May 16;80(23):2118–27.

Muanprasat C, Chatsudthipong V. Chitosan oligosaccharide: Biological activities and potential therapeutic applications. *Pharmacol Ther.* 2017 Feb;170:80–97.

Pittler MH, Ernst E. Dietary supplements for body-weight reduction: a systematic review. *Am J Clin Nutr.* 2004 Apr;79(4):529–36.

Ríos-Hoyo A, Gutiérrez-Salmeán G. New Dietary Supplements for Obesity: What We Currently Know. *Curr Obes Rep.* 2016 Jun;5(2):262–70.

Trivedi VR, Satia MC, Deschamps A, *et al.* Single-blind, placebo controlled randomised clinical study of chitosan for body weight reduction. *Nutr J.* 2016 Jan 8;15(1):3. doi: 10.1186/s12937–016–0122–8.

GINGER

Baliga MS, Haniadka R, Pereira MM, et al. Update on the chemopreventive effects of ginger and its phytochemicals. *Crit Rev Food Sci Nutr.* 2011 Jul;51(6):499–523.

Dugasani S, Pichika MR, Nadarajah VD, et al. Comparative antioxidant and anti-inflammatory effects of [6]-gingerol,[8]-gingerol, [10]-gingerol and [6]-shogaol. *J Ethnopharmacol.* 2010 Feb 3;127(2):515–20.

Lee DH, Kim DW, Jung CH, Lee YJ, Park D. Gingerol sensitizes TRAIL-induced apoptotic cell death of glioblastoma cells. *Toxicol Appl Pharmacol.* 2014 Sep 15;279(3):253–65.

Liju VB, Jeena K, Kuttan R. Gastroprotective activity of essential oils from turmeric and ginger. *J Basic Clin Phsiol Pharmacol.*2015 Jan;26(1):95–103.

Ryan JL, Heckler CE, Roscoe JA, et al. Ginger (*Zingiber officinale*) reduces acute chemotherapy-induced nausea: A URCC CCOP study of 576 patients. *Supportive Care in Cancer.* 2012;20(7):1479–1489.

Sang S, Hong J, Wu H, et al. Increased growth inhibitory effects on human cancer cells and anti-inflammatory potency of shogaols from Zingiber officinale relative to gingerols. *J Agric Food Chem.* 2009 Nov 25;57(22):10645–50.

GINKGO

Amieva H, Meillon C, Helmer C, Barberger-Gateau P, Dartigues JF. *Ginkgo biloba* extract and long-term cognitive decline: a 20-year follow-up population-based study. *PLoS One.* 2013 8(1), p.e52755.

Diamond BJ, Shiflett SC, Feiwel N, et al. *Ginkgo biloba* extract: mechanisms and clinical indications. *Archives of Physical Medicine and Rehabilitation.* 2000 81(5), pp.668–678.

Kanowski S, Herrmann WM, Stephan K, Wierich W, Hörr, R. Proof of efficacy of the *ginkgo biloba* special extract EGb 761 in outpatients suffering from mild to moderate primary degenerative dementia of the Alzheimer type or multi-infarct dementia. *Pharmacopsychiatry.* 1996 29(02), pp.47–56.

Le Bars PL, Katz MM, Berman N, et al. A placebo-controlled, double-blind, randomized trial of an extract of *Ginkgo biloba* for dementia. *JAMA.* 1997 278(16), pp.1327–1332.

GINSENG

Barton DL, Liu H, Dakhil SR, Linquist B, et al. Wisconsin Ginseng (*Panax quinquefolius*) to improve cancer-related fatigue: a randomized, double-blind trial, N07C2. *J Natl Cancer Inst.* 2013 Aug 21;105(16):1230–8.

Hong B, Ji YH, Hong JH, Nam KY, Ahn TY. A double-blind crossover study evaluating the efficacy of Korean red ginseng in patients with erectile dysfunction: a preliminary report. *J Urol.* 2002 Nov;168(5):2070–3.

Hong M, Lee YH, Kim S, et al. Anti-inflammatory and antifatigue effect of Korean Red Ginseng in patients with nonalcoholic fatty liver disease. *J Ginseng Res.* 2016 Jul;40(3):203–10.

Im K, Kim J, Min H. Ginseng, the natural effectual antiviral: Protective effects of Korean

Red Ginseng against viral infection. *J Ginseng Res.* 2016 Oct;40(4):309–314.

Kim DS, Kim Y, Jeon JY, Kim MG. Effect of Red Ginseng on cytochrome P450 and P-glycoprotein activities in healthy volunteers. *J Ginseng Res.* 2016 Oct;40(4):375–381.

Kim HG, Cho JH, Yoo SR, et al. Antifatigue effects of *Panax ginseng* C.A. Meyer: a randomised, double-blind, placebo-controlled trial. *PLoS One.* 2013 Apr 17;8(4):e61271.

Nguyen CT, Luong TT, Lee SY, et al. Panax ginseng aqueous extract prevents pneumococcal sepsis in vivo by potentiating cell survival and diminishing inflammation. *Phytomedicine.* 2015 Oct 15;22(11):1055–61.

Oh KJ, Chae MJ, Lee HS, Hong HD, Park K. Effects of Korean red ginseng on sexual arousal in menopausal women: placebo-controlled, double-blind crossover clinical study. *J Sex Med.* 2010 Apr;7(4 Pt 1):1469–77.

Oliynyk S, Oh S. Actoprotective effect of ginseng: improving mental and physical performance. *J Ginseng Res.* 2013 Apr;37(2):144–66.

Reay JL, Kennedy DO, Scholey AB. Effects of *Panax ginseng,* consumed with and without glucose, on blood glucose levels and cognitive performance during sustained 'mentally demanding' tasks. *J Psychopharmacol.* 2006 Nov;20(6):771–81.

Reay JL, Kennedy DO, Scholey AB. Single doses of *Panax ginseng* (G115) reduce blood glucose levels and improve cognitive performance during sustained mental activity. *J Psychopharmacol.* 2005 Jul;19(4):357–65.

Reay JL, Scholey AB, Kennedy DO. *Panax ginseng* (G115) improves aspects of working memory performance and subjective ratings of calmness in healthy young adults. *Hum Psychopharmacol.* 2010 Aug;25(6):462–71.

Tang X, Gan XT, Rajapurohitam V, et al. North American ginseng (*Panax quinquefolius*) suppresses [beta]-adrenergic-dependent signalling, hypertrophy, and cardiac dysfunction. *Can J Physiol Pharmacol.* 2016 Aug 17:1–11.

Yennurajalingam S, Reddy A, Tannir NM, et al. High-Dose Asian Ginseng (*Panax Ginseng*) for Cancer-Related Fatigue: A Preliminary Report. *Integr Cancer Ther.* 2015 Sep;14(5):419–27.

GLUTATHIONE

Flanagan RJ, Meredith TJ. Use of N-acetylcysteine in clinical toxicology. *Am J Med.* 1991 Sep 30;91(3C):131S–139S.

Hinson JA, Roberts DW, James LP. Mechanisms of Acetaminophen-Induced Liver Necrosis. *Handb Exp Pharmacol.* 2010;196:369–405.

James SJ, et al. Cellular and mitochondrial glutathione redox imbalance in lymphoblastoid cells derived from children with autism. *FASEB J.* 2009 Aug;23(8):2374–2383.

Larson AM, et al. Acetaminophen-induced acute liver failure: Results of a United States multicenter, prospective study. *Hepatology.* 2005 Dec; 42(6): 1364–1372.

Lauterburg BH, Corcoran GB, Mitchell JR. Mechanism of Action of N-Acetylcysteine in the Protection Against the Hepatotoxicity of Acetaminophen in Rats In Vivo. *J Clin Invest.* 1983 Apr;71(4):980–991.

Martensson J, Meister A. Glutathione deficiency decreases tissue ascorbate levels in newborn rats: ascorbate spares glutathione and protects. *PNAS.* 1991 Jun;88(11):4656–4660.

Mirochnitchenko O, Weisbrot-Lefkowitz M, Reuhl K, Chen L, Yang C, Inouye M. Acetaminophen Toxicity. Opposite effects of two forms of glutathione peroxidase. *J Biol Chem.* 1999 Apr 9;274(15):10349–10355.

Paolisso G, Tagliamonte MR, Rizzo MR, Manzella D, Gambardella A, Varricchio M. Oxidative Stress and Advancing Age: Results in Healthy Centenarians. *Journal of the American Geriatrics Society.* 1998 July; 46(7):833–838.

Rose S, et al. Evidence of oxidative damage and inflammation associated with low glutathione redox status in the autism brain. *Transl Psychiatry.* 2012 Jul 10;2:e134.

Sachi G, et al. Reduced intravenous glutathione in the treatment of early Parkinson's disease. *Prog Neuropsychopharmacol Biol Psychiatry.* 1996 Oct;20(7):1159–1170.

Schmitt B, Vicenzi M, Garrel C, Denis FM. Effects of N-acetylcysteine, oral glutathione (GSH) and a novel sublingual form of GSH on oxidative stress markers: A comparative crossover study. *Redox Biology.* 2015;6:198–205.

Sumiyoshi Y, Hashine K, Kasahara K, Karashima T. Glutathione chemoprotection therapy against CDDP-induced neurotoxicity in patients with invasive bladder cancer. [Article in Japanese]. *Gan To Kagaku Ryoho.* 1996 Sep;23(11): 1506–1508.

GRAPE SEED EXTRACT

Asha Devi S, et al. Grape seed proanthocyanidin lowers brain oxidative stress in adult and middle-aged rats. *Exp Gerontol.* 2011 Nov;46(11):958–64.

Badavi M, Abedi HA, Sarkaki AR, Dianat M. Co-administration of Grape Seed Extract and Exercise Training Improves Endothelial Dysfunction of Coronary Vascular Bed of STZ-Induced Diabetic Rats. *Iran Red Crescent Med J.* 2013 Oct;15(10):e7624.

Belcaro G, et al. Grape seed procyanidins in pre- and mild hypertension: a registry study. *Evid Based Complement Alternat Med.* 2013;2013:313142.

Crane PK, Walker R, Hubbard RA, et al. Glucose levels and risk of dementia. *N Engl J Med.* 2013 Aug 8;369(6):540–8.

Derry M, et al. Differential effects of grape seed extract against human colorectal cancer cell lines: The intricate role of death receptors and mitochondria. *Cancer Lett.* 2012 Dec 23. pii: S0304–3835(12)00732-X.

Ding Y, et al. Proanthocyanidins protect against early diabetic peripheral neuropathy by modulating endoplasmic reticulum stress. *J Nutr Biochem.* 2014 Jul;25(7):765–72.

Dinicola S, et al. Antiproliferative and apoptotic effects triggered by Grape Seed Extract (GSE) versus epigallocatechin and procyanidins on colon cancer cell lines. *Int J Mol Sci.* 2012;13(1):651–64.

Kaur M, Agarwal C, Agarwal R. Anticancer and cancer chemopreventive potential of grape seed extract and other grape-based products. *J Nutr.* 2009 Sep;139(9):1806S-12S.

Olas B, et al. The polyphenol-rich extract from grape seeds inhibits platelet signaling pathways triggered by both proteolytic and non-proteolytic agonists. *Platelets.* 2012;23(4):282–9.

Razavi SM, et al. Red grape seed extract improves lipid profiles and decreases oxidized low-density lipoprotein in patients with mild hyperlipidemia. *J Med Food.* 2013;16(3):255–8.

Sharma G, Tyagi AK, Singh RP, Chan DC, Agarwal R. Synergistic anti-cancer effects of grape seed extract and conventional cytotoxic agent doxorubicin against human breast carcinoma cells. *Breast Cancer Res Treat.* 2004 May;85(1):1–12.

Veluri R, et al. Fractionation of grape seed extract and identification of gallic acid as one of the major active constituents causing growth inhibition and apoptotic death of DU145 human prostate carcinoma cells. *Carcinogenesis.* 2006 Jul;27(7):1445–53.

Zhang Y, et al. Antithrombotic effect of grape seed proanthocyanidins extract in a rat model of deep vein thrombosis. *J Vasc Surg.* 2011;53(3):743–53.

GREEN TEA

Arab H, Mahjoub S, Hajian-Tilaki K, Moghadasi M. The effect of green tea consumption on oxidative stress markers and cognitive function in patients with Alzheimer's disease: A prospective intervention study. *Caspian J Intern Med*. 2016 Summer;7(3):188–194.

Bettuzzi S, Brausi M, Rizzi F, Castagnetti G, Peraccbia G, Corti A. Chemo prevention of human prostate cancer by oral administration of green tea catechins in volunteers with high-grade prostate intraepithelial neoplasia: a preliminary report from a one-year proof-of-principle study. *Canctr Res*. 2006;66:1234–1240.

Cai X, Campbell N, Khan B, Callahan C, Boustani M. Long-term anticholinergic use and the aging brain. *Alzheimers Dement*. 2013;9(4):377–385.

Cardoso GA, Salgado JM, Cesar Mde C, Donado-Pestana CM. The effects of green tea consumption and resistance training on body composition and resting metabolic rate in overweight or obese women. *J Med Food*. 2013 Feb;16(2):120–7.

Chen IJ, Liu CY, Chiu JP, Hsu CH. Therapeutic effect of high-dose green tea extract on weight reduction: A randomized, double-blind, placebo-controlled clinical trial. *Clin Nutr*. 2016 Jun;35(3):592–9.

Fox C, Smith T, Maidment I, et al. Effect of medications with anti-cholinergic properties on cognitive function, delirium, physical function and mortality: a systematic review. *Age Ageing*. 2014 Sep;43(5):604–15.

Gray SL, Anderson ML, Dublin S, et al. Cumulative use of strong anticholinergics and incident dementia: a prospective cohort study. *JAMA Intern Med*. 2015 Mar;175(3):401–7. doi: 10.1001/jamainternmed.2014.7663.

Janssens PL, Hursel R, Westerterp-Plantenga MS. Nutraceuticals for body-weight management: The role of green tea catechins. *Physiol Behav*. 2016 Aug 1;162:83–7.

Khan N, Adhami VM, Mukhtar H. Review: green tea polyphenols in chemoprevention of prostate cancer: preclinical and clinical studies. *Nutr Cancer*. 2009 Nov;61(6):836–41.

Kim HK, Kim M, Kim S, Kim M, Chung JH. Effects of green tea polyphenol on cognitive and acetylcholinesterase activities. *Biosci Biotechnol Biochem*. 2004 Sep;68(9):1977–9.

Kurahashi N, Sasazuki S, Iwasaki M, Inoue M, Tsugane S. Green tea consumption and prostate cancer risk in Japanese men: a prospoctive study. *Am J Epidemiol*. 2008;167:71–77.

Kuriyama S, Shimazu T, Ohmori K, Kikuchi N, Nakaya N, Nishino Y, Tsubono Y, Tsuji I. Green tea consumption and mortality due to cardiovascular disease, cancer, and all causes in Japan: the Ohsaki study. *JAMA*. 2006;296(10):1255–65.

Kuriyama S. The relation between green tea consumption and cardiovascular disease as evidenced by epidemiological studies. *J Nutr*. 2008 Aug;138(8):1548S–1553S.

Li G, Zhang Y, Thabane L, Mbuagbaw L, Liu A, Levine MA, Holbrook A. Effect of green tea supplementation on blood pressure among overweight and obese adults: a systematic review and meta-analysis. *J Hypertens*. 2015 Feb;33(2):243–54.

Lihn AS, Pedersen SB, Richelsen B. Adiponectin: action, regulation and association to insulin sensitivity. *Obes Rev*. 2005 Feb;6(1):13–21.

Liu J, Sun Y, Zhang H, et al. Theanine from tea and its semi-synthetic derivative TBrC suppress human cervical cancer growth and migration by inhibiting EGFR/Met-Akt/NF-[kappa]B signaling. *Eur J Pharmacol*. 2016 Sep 6;791:297–307.

Schliebs R, Arendt T. The cholinergic system in aging and neuronal degeneration. *Behav Brain*

Res. 2011 Aug 10;221(2):555–63. doi: 10.1016/j. bbr.2010.11.058. Epub 2010 Dec 9.

Siddiqui IA, Saleem M, Adhami VM, Asim M, Mukhtar H. Tea beverage in chemoprevention and chemotherapy of prostate cancer. *Acta Pharmacol Sin.* 2007 Sep;28(9):1392–408.

Suzuki T, Pervin M, Goto S, Isemura M, Nakamura Y. Beneficial Effects of Tea and the Green Tea Catechin Epigallocatechin-3-gallate on Obesity. *Molecules.* 2016 Sep 29;21(10).

Thangapazham RL, Singh AK, Sharma A, Warren J, Gaddipati JP, Maheshwari RK. Green tea polyphenols and its constituent epigallocatechin gallate inhibits proliferation of human breast cancer cells in vitro and in vivo. *Cancer Lett.* 2007;245(1–2):232–41.

Wang P, Henning SM, Magyar CE, Elshimali Y, Heber D, Vadgama JV. Green tea and quercetin sensitize PC-3 xenograft prostate tumors to docetaxel chemotherapy. *J Exp Clin Cancer Res.* 2016 May 6;35:73.

HAWTHORN

"Crataegus." *Merriam-Webster*.com. 2016. Web. 22 Nov. 2016. http://www.merriam-webster.com.

Asgary S, Naderi GH, Sadeghi M, Kelishadi R, Amiri M. Antihypertensive effect of Iranian Crataegus curvisepala Lind.: a randomized, double-blind study. *Drugs Exp Clin Res.* 2004;30(5–8):221–225.

Degenring FH, Suter A, Weber M, Saller R. A randomised double blind placebo controlled clinical trial of a standardized extract of fresh Crataegus berries (Crataegisan) in the treatment of patients with congestive heart failure NYHA II. *Phytomedicine.* 2003;10(5):363–369.

Heidenreich PA, et al. Forecasting the Future of Cardiovascular Disease in the United States. *Circulation.* 2011;123:933–944.

Hull KH. *Indiana Medical History Museum:*

Guide to the Medicinal Plant Garden. Indianapolis: Indiana Medical History Museum, 2010. Web. 22 Nov. 2016. http://www.imhm.org/resources/documents/binder1_mpg_guide_2010_sfs.pdf

Orhan IE. Phytochemical and pharmacological activity profile of Crataegus oxyacantha L. (hawthorn)—A cardiotonic herb. *Curr Med Chem.* 2016 Sep 18. [Epub ahead of print].

Pittler MH, Schmidt K, Ernst E. Hawthorn extract for treating chronic heart failure: meta-analysis of randomized trials. *Am J Med.* 2003 Jun 1;114(8):665–674.

Rezaei-Golmisheh A, Malekinejad H, Asri-Rezaei S, Farshid AA, Akbari P. Hawthorn ethanolic extracts with triterpenoids and flavonoids exert hepatoprotective effects and suppress the hypercholesterolemia-induced oxidative stress in rats. *Iran J Basic Med Sci.* 2015 Jul;18(7):691–699.

Tassell MC, Kingston R, Gilroy D, Lehane M, Furey A. Hawthorn (*Crataegus* spp.) in the treatment of cardiovascular disease. *Pharmacogn Rev.* 2010 Jan-Jun;4(7):32–41.

Walker AF, et al. Hypotensive effects of hawthorn for patients with diabetes taking prescription drugs: a randomised controlled trial. *Br J Gen Pract.* 2006 Jun;56(527):437–443.

Walker AF, Marakis G, Morris AP, Robinson PA. Promising hypotensive effect of hawthorn extract: a randomized double-blind pilot study of mild, essential hypertension. *Phytother Res.* 2002 Feb;16(1):48–54.

HEMP OIL

Welty TE, Luebke A, Gidal BE. Cannabidiol: promise and pitfalls. *Epilepsy Curr.* 2014 Sep;14(5):250–252.

Rabinski, G. "Understanding Cannabinoid Receptors: Why Cannabis Affects Humans," November 19, 2015. Available at: https://

www.massroots.com/learn/what-are-canna binoid-receptors.

La Porta C, Bura SA, Llorente-Onaindia J, *et al.* Role of the endocannabinoid system in the emotional manifestations of osteoarthritis pain. *Pain.* 2015 Oct;156(10):2001–12.

Cunha JM, Carlini EA, Pereira AE, Ramos OL, Pimentel C, Gagliardi R, Sanvito WL, Lander N, Mechoulam R. Chronic administration of cannabidiol to healthy volunteers and epileptic patients. *Pharmacology.* 1980;21:175–185.

Tzadok M, Uliel-Siboni S, Linder I, *et al.* CBD-enriched medical cannabis for intractable pediatric epilepsy: The current Israeli experience. *Seizure.* 2016 Feb;35:41–4.

Karniol I.G., Shirakawa I., Kasinski N., Pfeferman A., Carlini E.A. Cannabidiol interferes with the effects of delta 9-tetrahydrocannabinol in man. *Eur. J. Pharmacol.* 1974;28:172–177.

Zuardi A.W., Shirakawa I., Finkelfarb E., Karniol I.G. Action of cannabidiol on the anxiety and other effects produced by delta 9-THC in normal subjects. *Psychopharmacology* (Berl.) 1982;76:245–250.

Richardson D, Pearson RG, Kurian N, *et al.* Characterisation of the cannabinoid receptor system in synovial tissue and fluid in patients with osteoarthritis and rheumatoid arthritis. *Arthritis Res Ther.* 2008;10(2):R43.

La Porta C, Bura SA, Llorente-Onaindia J, *et al.* Role of the endocannabinoid system in the emotional manifestations of osteoarthritis pain. *Pain.* 2015 Oct;156(10):2001–12.

Lynch ME, Cesar-Rittenberg P, Hohmann AG. A double-blind, placebo-controlled, crossover pilot trial with extension using an oral mucosal cannabinoid extract for treatment of chemotherapy-induced neuropathic pain. *J Pain Symptom Manage.* 2014 Jan;47(1):166–73.

Serpell M, Ratcliffe S, Hovorka J, *et al.* A double-blind, randomized, placebo-controlled, parallel group study of THC/CBD spray in peripheral neuropathic pain treatment. *Eur J Pain.* 2014 Aug;18(7):999-1012. doi: 10.1002/j.1532-2149.2013.00445.x. Epub 2014 Jan 13.

Hoggart B, Ratcliffe S, Ehler E, *et al.* A multicentre, open-label, follow-on study to assess the long-term maintenance of effect, tolerance and safety of THC/CBD oromucosal spray in the management of neuropathic pain. *J Neurol.* 2015 Jan;262(1):27–40.

Patti F, Messina S, Solaro C, *et al.* Efficacy and safety of cannabinoid oromucosal spray for multiple sclerosis spasticity. *J Neurol Neurosurg Psychiatry.* 2016 Sep;87(9):944–51.

Khan MI, Soboci ska AA, Czarnecka AM, Król M, Botta B, Szczylik C. The Therapeutic Aspects of the Endocannabinoid System (ECS) for Cancer and their Development: From Nature to Laboratory. *Curr Pharm Des.* 2016 Mar; 22(12): 1756–1766.

Ladin DA, Soliman E, Griffin L, Van Dross R. Preclinical and Clinical Assessment of Cannabinoids as Anti-Cancer Agents. *Front Pharmacol.* 2016 Oct 7;7:361. eCollection 2016.

Singer E, Judkins J, Salomonis N, *et al.* Reactive oxygen species-mediated therapeutic response and resistance in glioblastoma. *Cell Death Dis.* 2015 Jan 15;6:e1601.

Massi P, Valenti M, Vaccani A, Gasperi V, Perletti G, Marras E, *et al.* 5-Lipoxygenase and anandamide hydrolase (FAAH) mediate the antitumor activity of cannabidiol, a non-psychoactive cannabinoid. *J Neurochem* 2008; 104: 1091–1100.

McKallip RJ, Jia W, Schlomer J, Warren JW, Nagarkatti PS, Nagarkatti M. Cannabidiol-induced apoptosis in human leukemia cells: a novel role of cannabidiol in the regulation of p22phox and Nox4 expression. *Mol Pharmacol* 2006; 70: 897–908.

De Petrocellis L, Ligresti A, Schiano Moriello A, Iappelli M, Verde R, Stott CG *et al.* Non-THC cannabinoids inhibit prostate carcinoma growth *in vitro* and *in vivo*: pro-apoptotic effects and underlying mechanisms. *Br J Pharmacol* 2012; 168: 79–102

Kogan NM, Melamed E, Wasserman E, *et al*. Cannabidiol, a Major Non-Psychotropic Cannabis Constituent Enhances Fracture Healing and Stimulates Lysyl Hydroxylase Activity in Osteoblasts. *J Bone Miner Res*. 2015 Oct;30(10):1905–13.

Dobrosi N, Tóth BI, Nagy G, *et al*. Endocannabinoids enhance lipid synthesis and apoptosis of human sebocytes via cannabinoid receptor-2-mediated signaling. *FASEB J*. 2008 Oct;22(10):3685–95.

HINTONIA LATIFLORA

"At a Glance 2016: Diabetes." Centers for Disease Control and Prevention. Available at: http://www.cdc.gov/chronicdisease/resources/publications/aag/pdf/2016/diabetes-aag.pdf. Accessed: November 15, 2016.

Crane P, et al. Glucose levels and risk of dementia. *New Engl J Med*. 2013;369:540–548

Cristians S, Bye R, Navarrete A, Mata R. Gastroprotective effect of *Hintonia latiflora* and *Hintonia standleyana* aqueous extracts and compounds. *J Ethnopharmacol*. 2013 Jan 30;145(2):530–535.

Korecova M, Hladikova M. Treatment of mild and moderate type-2 diabetes: open prospective trial with *Hintonia latiflora* extract. *Eur J Med Res*. 2014 Mar 28;19:16.

Kuhr, R. Oral Diabetes Therapy with an Euphorbiacean Extract. *Der Landarzt*, 1953. 29(23):1–8.

Mata R, Cristians S, Escandón-Rivera S, Juárez-Reyes K, Rivero-Cruz I. Mexican antidiabetic herbs: valuable sources of inhibitors of [alpha] -glucosidases. *J Nat Prod*. 2013 Mar 22;76(3):468–483.

Schmidt M, Hladikova M. Hintonia concen-trate—for the dietary treatment of increased blood sugar values: Results of a multicentric, prospective, non-interventional study with a defined dry concentrate of hintonia latiflora. *Naturheilpraxis*. Feb. 2014. (Translated article).

Schmidt M, Hladikova M. Hintonia concen-trate—for the dietary treatment of increased blood sugar values: Results of a multicentric, prospective, non-interventional study with a defined dry concentrate of *Hintonia latiflora*. *Naturheilpraxis*. Feb. 2014. (Translated article).

Vierling C, Baumgartner CM, Bollerhey M, et al. The vasodilating effect of a *Hintonia latiflora* extract with antidiabetic action. *Phytomedicine*. 2014 Oct 15;21(12):1582–86.

HOLY BASIL

Archana R, Namasivayam A. Effect of Ocimum sanctum on noise induced changes in neutrophil functions. *Journal of Ethnopharmacology*. 73, no. 1 (2000): 81–85.

Bhargava KP, Singh N. "Anti-stress activity of *Ocimum sanctum Linn*." *The Indian Journal of Medical Research*. 73 (1981): 443.

Gupta, SK, Prakash J, Srivastava S. Validation of traditional claim of Tulsi, *Ocimum sanctum Linn*. as a medicinal plant. *Indian Journal of Experimental Biology* 40, no. 7 (2002): 765–773.

Opendak M, Gould E. Adult neurogenesis: a substrate for experience-dependent change. *Trends in Cognitive Sciences*. 19, no. 3 (2015): 151–161.

Sampath S, Mahapatra SC, Padhi MM, Sharma R, Talwar A. Holy basil (*Ocimum sanctum Linn*.) leaf extract enhances specific cognitive parameters in healthy adult volunteers: A placebo controlled study. *Indian J Physiol Pharmacol*. 2015 Jan-Mar;59(1):69–77.

Samson J, Sheeladevi R, Ravindran R. Oxidative stress in brain and antioxidant activity of

Ocimum sanctum in noise exposure. *Neurotoxicology*. 28, no. 3 (2007): 679–685.

Sembulingam K, Sembulingam P, Namasivayam A. Effect of *Ocimum sanctum Linn* on the changes in central cholinergic system induced by acute noise stress. *Journal of Ethnopharmacology*. 96, no. 3 (2005): 477–482.

IODINE

Abraham, G.E. The History of Iodine in Medicine Part III: Thyroid Fixation and Medical Iodophobia. *Original Internist*. 2006;13: 71–78.

Cann SA, van Netten JP, van Netten C. Hypothesis: iodine, selenium and the development of breast cancer. *Cancer Causes Control*. 2000 Feb;11(2):121–7.

Ghent WR, Eskin BA, Low DA, Hill LP. Iodine replacement in fibrocystic disease of the breast. *Can J Surg*. 1993 Oct;36(5):453–60.

Patrick L. Iodine: deficiency and therapeutic considerations. *Altern Med Rev*. 2008 Jun;13(2):116–27.

Reinhardt W, Kohl S, Hollmann D, et al. Efficacy and safety of iodine in the postpartum period in an area of mild iodine deficiency. *Eur J Med Res*. 1998;3(4):203–10.

Stoddard FR 2nd, Brooks AD, Eskin BA, Johannes GJ. Iodine alters gene expression in the MCF7 breast cancer cell line: evidence for an anti-estrogen effect of iodine. *Int J Med Sci*. 2008 Jul 8;5(4):189–96.

Triggiani V, Tafaro E, Giagulli VA, et al. Role of iodine, selenium and other micronutrients in thyroid function and disorders. *Endocr Metab Immune Disord Drug Targets*. 2009;9(3):277–94.

IODINE RECOMMENDED READING

Brownstein, David, M.D. *Iodine: Why You Need It, Why You Can't Live Without It* (Medical Alternatives Press, 2009).

MELISSA

Abate G, et al. Controlled multicenter study on the therapeutic effectiveness of mesoglycan in patients with cerebrovascular disease. [Article in Italian]. *Minerva Med*. 1991 Mar;82(3):101–105.

Andreozzi GM. Effectiveness of mesoglycan in patients with previous deep venous thrombosis and chronic venous insufficiency. *Minerva Cardioangiol*. 2007 Dec;55(6):741–753.

Awad R, Muhammad A, Durst T, Trudeau VL, Arnason JT. Bioassay-guided fractionation of lemon balm (*Melissa officinalis L.*) using an in vitro measure of GABA transaminase activity. *Phytother Res*. 2009 Aug;23(8):1075–81.

Cases J, Ibarra A, Feuillère N, Roller M, Sukkar SG. Pilot trial of *Melissa officinalis* L. leaf extract in the treatment of volunteers suffering from mild-to-moderate anxiety disorders and sleep disturbances. *Med J Nutrition Metab*. 2011 Dec;4(3):211–218.

Coresh J, Selvin E, Stevens LA. Prevalence of Chronic Kidney Disease in the United States. *JAMA*. 2007;298(17):2038–2047.

Di Base A. Mesoglycan treatment in Raynaud phenomenon: a case series. *Minerva Cardioangiol*. 2013 Jun;61(3):323–331.

Donnell R, Emslie-Smith AM, Gardner ID, Morris AD. Vascular complications of diabetes. *BMJ*. 2000 Apr 15;320(7241):1062–1066.

Giorgetti PL, Marenghi MC, Bianciardi P. Heparan sulfate in the therapy of postphlebitic syndrome. Evaluation of the efficacy and tolerability as compared to mesoglycan. [Article in Italian]. *Minerva Cardioangiol*. 1997 Jun;45(6):279–284.

Haffner SM. Coronary Heart Disease in Patients with Diabetes. *N Engl J Med*. 2000 Apr 6;342:1040–1042.

Heinrich PA, et al. Forecasting the Future of

Cardiovascular Disease in the United States. *Circulation.* 2011;123:933–944.

Kennedy DO, Wake G, Savelev S, et al. Modulation of mood and cognitive performance following acute administration of single doses of *Melissa officinalis* (Lemon balm) with human CNS nicotinic and muscarinic receptor-binding properties. *Neuropsychopharmacology.* 2003 Oct;28(10):1871–81.

Laurora G, et al. Control of the progress of arteriosclerosis in high risk subjects treated with mesoglycan. Measuring the intima media [Article in Italian]. *Minerva Cardioangiol.* 1998 Mar;46(3):41–47.

Maresca L, Foggia C, Leonardo G. Restoring microvascular efficiency with mesoglycan in women affected by moderate chronic venous disease. *Minerva Cardioangiol.* 2015 Apr;63(2):105–111.

MESOGLYCAN

Nenci GG, et al. Treatment of intermittent claudication with mesoglycan—a placebo-controlled, double-blind study. *Thromb Haemost.* 2001 Nov; 86(5):1181–1187.

Pacella E, et al. A pilot clinical study on the effectiveness of mesoglycan against diabetic retinopathy. *Clin Ter.* 2012;163(1):19–22.

Petruzzellis V & Velon A. Therapeutic action of oral mesoglycan in the pharmacologic treatment of the varicose syndrome and its complications. [Article in Italian]. *Minerva Med.* 1985 Mar 24;76(12):543–548.

Villani T, Scarselli M, Pieri A, Gatti M, Santini M, Pasquetti P. Pharmacological treatment of mechanical edema: a randomized controlled trial about the effects of mesoglycan. *Eur J Phys Rehabil Med.* 2009 Mar;45(1):21–29.

Zarei A, Changizi-Ashtiyani S, Taheri S, Hosseini N. A Brief Overview of the Effects of *Melissa officinalis L.* Extract on the Function of Various Body Organs. *Zahedan Journal of Research in Medical Sciences.* 2014.

MYRTLE

Ebrahimabadi EH, Ghoreishi SM, Masoum S, Ebrahimabadi AH. Combination of GC/FID/Mass spectrometry fingerprints and multivariate calibration techniques for recognition of antimicrobial constituents of *Myrtus communis* L. essential oil. *Journal of Chromatography B.* 2016 1008: 50–57.

Kehrl, W, Uwe S, Uwe D. Therapy for Acute Nonpurulent Rhinosinusitis with Cineole: Results of a Double-Blind, Randomized, Placebo-Controlled Trial. *The Laryngoscope* 2004 114, no. 4 : 738–742.

Matthys H, Christian M, Christian C, et al. Efficacy and tolerability of myrtol standardized in acute bronchitis. *Arzneimittelforschung.* 2000 50, no. 08: 700–711.

Mimica-Dukić N, Dušan B, Slavenko G, et al. Essential oil of *Myrtus communis L.* as a potential antioxidant and antimutagenic agents. *Molecules* 2010 15, no. 4: 2759–2770.

Tesche S, Frank M, Uwe S, Jan-Christian E, Uwe D. The value of herbal medicines in the treatment of acute non-purulent rhinosinusitis. *European Archives of Oto-Rhino-Laryngology.* 2008 265, no. 11 2008: 1355–1359.

OLIVE

Boss A, et al. Human Intervention Study to Assess the Effects of Supplementation with Olive Leaf Extract on Peripheral Blood Mononuclear Cell Gene Expression. *Int J Mol Sci.* 2016 Dec 2;17(12). Pii: E2019.

de Bock, M et al. Human absorption and metabolism of oleuropein and hydroxytyrosol ingested as olive (*Olea europaea L.*)

leaf extract. *Food & Function*. November 2013;57(11):2079–2085.

Hernaez A, et al. Mediterranean Diet Improves High-Density Lipoprotein Function in High-Cardiovascular-Risk Individuals: A Randomized Controlled Trial. *Circulation*. 2017 Feb 14;135(7):633–643.

Lockyer S, Corona G, Yagoob P, Spencer JP, Rowland I. Secoiridoids delivered as olive leaf extract induce acute improvements in human vascular function and reduction of an inflammatory cytokine: a randomised, double-blind, placebo-controlled, cross-over trial. *Br J Nutr*. 2015 Jul 14;114(1):75–83.

Susalit E, Agus N, Tjandrawinata RR, Nofiarny D, Perrinjaguet-Moccetti T, Verbruggen M. Olive (Olea europaea) leaf extract effective in patients with stage-1 hypertension: comparison with Captopril. Phytomedicine. 2011 Feb 15;18(4):251–258.

Talhaoui N, Taamalli A, Gomez-Caravaca AM, Fernandez-Gutierrez A, Segura-Carretero A. Phenolic compounds in olive leaves: Analytical determination, biotic and abiotic influence, and health benefits. *Food Research International*. November 2015;77(2)

OMEGA-3 FATTY ACIDS

Florent S, Malaplate-Armand C, Youssef I, et al. Docosahexaenoic acid prevents neuronal apoptosis induced by soluble amyloid-beta oligomers. *J Neurochem*. 2006 Jan;96(2):385–395.

Jones PJ, Demonty I, Chan YM, et al. Fish-oil esters of plant sterols differ from vegetable-oil sterol esters in triglycerides lowering, carotenoid bioavailability and impact on plasminogen activator inhibitor-1 (PAI-1) concentrations in hypercholesterolemic subjects. *Lipids Health Dis*. 2007 Oct 25;6:28.

Karalis DG. A Review of Clinical Practice Guidelines for the Management of Hypertriglyceridemia: A Focus on High Dose Omega-3 Fatty Acids. *Adv Ther*. 2017 Feb;34(2):300–323.

Liu JJ, Galfalvy HC, Cooper TB, et al. Omega-3 polyunsaturated fatty acid (PUFA) status in major depressive disorder with comorbid anxiety disorders. *J Clin Psychiatry*. 2013 Jul;74(7):732–738.

Parmentier M, Mahmoud CA, Linder M, Fanni J. Polar lipids: n-3 PUFA carriers for membranes and brain: nutritional interest and emerging processes. Oléagineux, Corps gras, *Lipides*. 2007 May 1;14(3–4):224–229.

Rondanelli M, Giacosa A, Opizzi A, et al. Long-chain Omega-3 polyunsaturated fatty acids supplementation in the treatment of elderly depression: effects on depressive symptoms, on phospholipids fatty acids profile and on health-related quality of life. *J Nutr Health Aging*. 2011 Jan; 15(1):37–44.

OREGANO

Bharti V, Vasudeva N, Sharma S, Duhan JS. Antibacterial activities of *Origanum vulgare* alone and in combination with different antimicrobials against clinical isolates of *Salmonella typhi*. Anc Sci Life. 2013 Apr;32(4):212–216.

Bouhdid S, Abrini J, Zhiri A, Espuny MJ, Manresa A. Investigation of functional and morphological changes in Pseudomonas aeruginosa and Staphylococcus aureus cells induced by *Origanum compactum* essential oil. *J Appl Microbiol*. 2009 May;106(5):1558–568.

Bouhdid S, Skali S N, Idaomar M. Antibacterial and antioxidant activities of *Origanum compactum* essential oil. *African J Biotech*. 2008;7(10): 1563–570.

Chaouki W, Leger DY, Eljastimi J, Beneytout JL, Hmamouchi M. Antiproliferative effect of extracts from *Aristolochia baetica* and *Origanum compactum* on human breast cancer cell line MCF-7. *Pharm Biol*. 2010 Mar;48(3):269–274.

Mayaud L, Carricajo A, Zhiri A, Aubert G. Comparison of bacteriostatic and bactericidal activity of 13 essential oils against strains with varying sensitivity to antibiotics. *Lett Appl Microbiol.* 2008;47(3):167–173.

Pesavento G, Maggini V, Maida I, *et al.* Essential Oil from *Origanum vulgare* Completely Inhibits the Growth of Multidrug-Resistant Cystic Fibrosis Pathogens. *Nat Prod Commun.* 2016 Jun;11(6):861–864.

Preuss HG, Echard B, Dadgar A, et al. Effects of Essential Oils and Monolaurin on Staphylococcus aureus: In Vitro and In Vivo Studies. *Toxicol Mech Methods.* 2005;15(4):279–285.

POMEGRANATE

Adhami VM, Khan N, and Mukhtar H. Cancer chemoprevention by pomegranate: laboratory and clinical evidence. *Nutrition and Cancer.* 2009. *61*(6), 811–815.

Grossmann ME, Mizuno NK, Schuster T, Cleary MP. 2010. Punicic acid is a ω-5 fatty acid capable of inhibiting breast cancer proliferation. *International Journal of Oncology.* 2010. *36*(2), 421.

Kim ND, Mehta R, Yu W, et al. Chemopreventive and adjuvant therapeutic potential of pomegranate (*Punica granatum*) for human breast cancer. *Breast Cancer Research and Treatment.* 2002. *71*(3), 203–217.

PROBIOTICS

Bixquert Jiménez M. Treatment of irritable bowel syndrome with probiotics. An etiopathogenic approach at last? *Rev Esp Enferm Dig.* 2009;101(8):553–564.

Ducrotté P, Sawant P, Jayanthi V. Clinical trial: *Lactobacillus plantarum* 299v (DSM 9843) improves symptoms of irritable bowel syndrome. *World J Gastroenterol.* 2012;18(30):4012–18.

Goossens D, Jonkers, D., Russel, et al. The effect of *Lactobacillus plantarum* 299v on the bacterial composition and metabolic activity in faeces of healthy volunteers: a placebo-controlled study on the onset and duration of effects. *Aliment Pharmacol Ther.* 2003;18(5):495–505.

Klarin, B., Johansson, M.L., Molin, G., Larsson, A. and Jeppsson, B.et al. Adhesion of the probiotic bacterium *Lactobacillus plantarum* 299v onto the gut mucosa in critically ill patients: a randomised open trial. *Crit Care.* 2005;9(3):R285–293

Michielan A, D'Incà R. Intestinal Permeability in Inflammatory Bowel Disease: Pathogenesis, Clinical Evaluation, and Therapy of Leaky Gut. *Mediators Inflamm.* 2015;2015:628157.

Niedzielin K, Kordecki H, Birkenfeld B. A controlled, double-blind, randomized study on the efficacy of *Lactobacillus plantarum* 299V in patients with irritable bowel syndrome. *Eur J Gastroenterol* Hepatol. 2001;13(10):1143–147.

Saez-Lara MJ, Gomez-Llorente C, Plaza-Diaz J, Gil A. The role of probiotic lactic acid bacteria and bifidobacteria in the prevention and treatment of inflammatory bowel disease and other related diseases: a systematic review of randomized human clinical trials. *Biomed Res Int.* 2015;2015:505878.

Wang W., Chen L., Zhou R., et al. Increased proportions of Bifidobacterium and the Lactobacillus group and loss of butyrate-producing bacteria in inflammatory bowel disease. *Journal of Clinical Microbiology.* 2014;52(2):398–406.

PROPOLIS

Astani A, Zimmermann S, Hassan E, et al. Antimicrobial activity of propolis special extract GH2002 against multidrug-resistant clinical isolates. *Pharmazie.* 2013 Aug: 68(8):695–701.

Castaldo S, Capasso F. Propolis, an old remedy used in modern medicine. *Fitoterapia,* (2002) 73, pp.S1–S6.

El-Shouny, W, Muagam, F, Sadik, Z, Walaa H. Antimicrobial Activity of Propolis Extract on URT Infections in Pediatric Patients Admitted to Al-Thowrah Hospital, Hodeidah City, Yemen. *World Journal of Medical Sciences*, (2012) 7(3), 172–177.

Hernandez-Reif M, Field T, Ironson G, Beutler J, Vera Y, Hurley J, et al.Natural killer cells and lymphocytes increase in women with breast cancer following massage therapy. *Int J Neurosci*. 2005 Apr; 115(4):495–510.

Huleihel, M.,Isanu V. Anti-herpes simplex virus effect of an aqueous extract of propolis. *The Israel Medical Association journal: IMAJ*, 2002 4 (11 Suppl), pp.923–927.

Khacha-Ananda S, Tragoolpua K., Chantawannakul P, Tragoolpua Y. Antioxidant and anti-cancer cell proliferation activity of propolis extracts from two extraction methods. *Asian Pacific Journal of Cancer Prevention*, 2013 14 (11):6991–6995.

Khayyal MT, El-Ghazaly MA, El-Khatib AS. Mechanisms involved in the anti-inflammatory effect of propolis extract. *Drugs under experimental and clinical research*. 1992 Dec;19(5):197–203.

Nolkemper S, Reichling J, Sensch KH,Schnitzler P. Mechanism of herpes simplex virus type 2 suppression by propolis extracts. *Phytomedicine*, (2010) 17(2), 132–138.

Sawicka D, Car H, Borawska MH, Nikliński J. The anticancer activity of propolis. *Folia Histochem Cytobiol*. 2012 Apr 24; 50(1):25–37.

PUMPKIN SEED EXTRACT

Bharti SK, Kumar A, Sharma NK, et al. Tocopherol from seeds of *Cucurbita pepo* against diabetes: validation by in vivo experiments supported by computational docking. *J Formos Med Assoc*. 2013 Nov;112(11):676–690.

El-Mosallamy AE, Sleem AA, Abdel-Salam OM, Shaffie N, Kenawy SA. Antihypertensive and cardioprotective effects of pumpkin seed oil. *J Med Food*. 2012 Feb;15(2):180–189.

Friederich M, Theurer C, Schlosser G. Prosta Fink Forte capsules in the treatment of benign prostatic hyperplasia. Multicentric surveillance study in 2245 patients. *Forsch Komplementarmed Klass Naturheilkd*. 2000;7:200–204.

Gossell-Williams M, Davis A, O'Connor N. Inhibition of testosterone-induced hyperplasia of the prostate of sprague-dawley rats by pumpkin seed oil. *J Med Food*. 2006 Summer;9(2):284–286.

Hong H, Kim CS, Maeng S. Effects of pumpkin seed oil and saw palmetto oil in Korean men with symptomatic benign prostatic hyperplasia. *Nutr Res Pract*. 2009 Winter;3(4):323–327.

Nishimura M, Ohkawara T, Sato H, Takeda H, Nishihira J. Pumpkin Seed Oil Extracted From Cucurbita maxima Improves Urinary Disorder in Human Overactive Bladder. *J Tradit Complement Med*. 2014 Jan;4(1):72–74.

Sogabe H, Terado T. Open clinical study of effects of pumpkin seed extract/soybean germ extract mixture-containing processed food on nocturia. *Jpn J Med Pharm Sci*. 2001 Nov;46(5):727–737.

Terado T et al. Elderly men with nocturnal pollakiuria: significant decrease of nightly urination frequency, improved quality of sleep, subjective improvement. *Jpn J Med Pharm Sci*. 2004; vol 52 (4).

Tsai YS, Tong YC, Cheng JT, Lee CH, Yang FS, Lee HY. Pumpkin seed oil and phytosterol-F can block testosterone/prazosin-induced prostate growth in rats. *Urol Int*. 2006;77(3):269–274.

RAVINTSARA

"Ravintsara versus Ravensara: What's the Difference?" Aromatic Studies. Available at: aromaticstudies.com/ravintsara-vs-ravensara

-whats-the-difference/. Accessed: February 21, 2017.

Costa R, Pizzimenti F, Marotta F, Dugo P, Santi L, Mondello L. Volatiles from steam-distilled leaves of some plant species from Madagascar and New Zealand and evaluation of their biological activity. *Nat Prod Commun.* 2010 Nov;5(11):1803–808.

Lee HJ, Hyun EA, Yoon WJ, et al. In vitro anti-inflammatory and anti-oxidative effects of Cinnamomum camphora extracts. *J Ethnopharmacol.* 2006 Jan 16;103(2):208–16. Epub 2005 Sep 22.

Marasini BP, Baral P, Aryal P, *et al.* Evaluation of antibacterial activity of some traditionally used medicinal plants against human pathogenic bacteria. *Biomed Res Int.* 2015;2015:265425.

Satyal P, Paudel P, Poudel A, Dosoky NS, Pokharel KK, Setzer WN. Bioactivities and compositional analyses of Cinnamomum essential oils from Nepal: C. *camphora, C. tamala,* and C. *glaucescens. Nat Prod Commun.* 2013 Dec;8(12):1777–784.

Singh P, Srivastava B, Kumar A, Dubey NK. Fungal contamination of raw materials of some herbal drugs and recommendation of *Cinnamomum camphora* oil as herbal fungitoxicant. *Microb Ecol.* 2008 Oct;56(3):555–560. Epub 2008 Mar 6.

RHODIOLA

Abidov M, Crendal F, Grachev S, Seifulla R, Ziegenfuss T. Effects of Extracts from *Rhodiola Rosea* and *Rhodiola Crenulata* (*Crassulaceae*) Roots on ATP Content in Mitochondria of Skeletal Muscles. *Bulletin of Experimental Biology and Medicine.* 2003;136(12):664–666.

Abidov M, Grachev S, Seifulla RD, Ziegenfuss TN. Extract of *Rhodiola rosea* Radix Reduces the Level of C-Reactive Protein and Creatinine Kinase in the Blood. *Bulletin of Experimental Biology and Medicine.* 2004;138(7):73–75.

Antonelli M, Kushner I. It's time to redefine inflammation. *FASEB J.* 2017 Feb 8. Epub ahead of print.

Bystritsky A, Kerwin L, Feusner JD. A pilot study of Rhodiola rosea (Rhodax) for generalized anxiety disorder (GAD). *J Altern Complement Med.* 2008 Mar;14(2):175–180.

Chex X, et al. Salidroside alleviates cachexia symptoms in mouse models of cancer cachexia via activation mTOR signaling. *J Cachexia Sarcopenia Muscle.* 2016 May;7(2):225–232.

Dallman MF, Pecoraro NC, la Fleur SE. Chronic stress and comfort foods: self-medication and abdominal obesity. *Brain, Behavior, and Immunity.* 2005;19(40:275–280.

De Bock K, Eijnde BO, Ramaekers M, Hespel P. Acute Rhodiola rosea intake can improve endurance exercise performance. *Int J Sport Nutr Exerc Metab.* 2004 Jun;14(3):298–307.

Diwaker D, Mishra KP, Ganju L, Singh SB. Rhodiola inhibits dengue virus multiplication by inducing innate immune response genes RIG-I, MDA5 and ISG in human monocytes. *Arch Virol.* 2014 Aug;159(8):1975–1986.

Fan XJ, Wang Y, Wang L, Zhu M. Salidroside induces apoptosis and autophagy in human colorectal cancer cells through inhibition of PI3K/Akt/mTOR pathway. *Oncol Rep.* 2016 Dec;36(6):3559–3567.

Fischer S, Doerr JM, Strahler J, Mewes R, Thieme K, Nater UM. Stress exacerbates pain in the everyday lives of women with fibromyalgia syndrome—The role of cortisol and alpha-amylase. *Psychoneuroendocrinology.* 2016 Jan;63:68–77.

Glaser R, Kiecolt-Glaser JK. Stress-associated immune modulation: relevance to viral infections and chronic fatigue syndrome. *The American Journal of Medicine.* 1998;105(3):35S–42S.

Olsson EM, von Scheele B, Panossian AG. A randomised, double-blind, placebo-controlled, parallel-group study of the stardardised extract shr-5 of the roots of Rhodiola rosea in the treatment of subjects with stress-related fatigue. *Planta Med.* 2009 Feb;75(2):105–112.

Orth-Gomer K, Wamala SP, Horsten M. Marital Stress Worsens Prognosis in Women With Coronary Heart Disease: The Stockholm Female Coronary Risk Study. *JAMA.* 2000;284(23):3008–3014.

Rosen RL, et al. Elevated C-reaction protein and posttraumatic stress pathology among survivors of the 9/11 World Trade Center attacks. *J Psychiatr Res.* 2017 Jan 16;89:14–21.

Zhao G, Shi A, Fan Z, Du Y. Salidroside inhibits the growth of human breast cancer in vitro and in vivo. *Oncol Rep.* 2015 May;33(5):2553–2560.

SAW PALMETTO

Geavlete P, Multescu R, Geavlete B. *Serenoa repens* extract in the treatment of benign prostatic hyperplasia. *Ther Adv Urol.* 2011 Aug;3(4):193–198.

Gerber GS, Kuznetsov D, Johnson BC, Burstein JD. Randomized, double-blind, placebo-controlled trial of saw palmetto in men with lower urinary tract symptoms. *Urology.* 2001 Dec;58(6):960–4; discussion 964–965.

Habib FK, Ross M, Ho CK, Lyons V, Chapman K. Serenoa repens (Permixon) inhibits the 5alpha-reductase activity of human prostate cancer cell lines without interfering with PSA expression. *Int J Cancer.* 2005 Mar 20;114(2):190–194.

Hong H, Kim CS, Maeng S. Effects of pumpkin seed oil and saw palmetto oil in Korean men with symptomatic benign prostatic hyperplasia. *Nutr Res Pract.* 2009 Winter;3(4):323–327.

Minutoli L, Bitto A, Squadrito F, *et al.* *Serenoa Repens*, lycopene and selenium: a triple therapeutic approach to manage benign prostatic hyperplasia. *Curr Med Chem.* 2013;20(10):1306–312.

Morgia G, Russo GI, Voce S, *et al.* *Serenoa repens*, lycopene and selenium versus tamsulosin for the treatment of LUTS/BPH. An Italian multicenter double-blinded randomized study between single or combination therapy (PROCOMB trial). *Prostate.* 2014 Nov;74(15):1471–480.

Russo A, Capogrosso P, La Croce G, *et al.* *Serenoa repens*, selenium and lycopene to manage lower urinary tract symptoms suggestive for benign prostatic hyperplasia. *Expert Opin Drug Saf.* 2016 Dec;15(12):1661–1670. Epub 2016 Jun 1.

Sökeland J. Combined sabal and urtica extract compared with finasteride in men with benign prostatic hyperplasia: analysis of prostate volume and therapeutic outcome. *BJU Int.* 2000 Sep;86(4):439–442.

SCHISANDRA

Chiu HF, Chen TY, Tzeng YT, Wang CK. Improvement of liver function in humans using a mixture of schisandra fruit extract and sesamin. *Phytother Res.* 2013 Mar;27(3):368–73.

Guo LY, Hung TM, Bae KH, et al. Anti-inflammatory effects of schisandrin isolated from the fruit of Schisandra chinensis Baill. *Eur J Pharmacol.* 2008;591(1–3):293–299

Panossian A, Wikman G. Pharmacology of Schisandra chinensis Bail.: an overview of Russian research and uses in medicine. *J Ethnopharmacol.* 2008 Jul 23;118(2):183–212.

Sun LJ, Wang GH, Wu B, et al. Effects of schisandra on the function of the pituitary-adrenal cortex, gonadal axis and carbohydrate metabolism in rats undergoing experimental chronic psychological stress, navigation and strenuous exercise. *Zhonghua Nan Ke Xue.* 2009;15(2):126–129.

SEA BUCKTHORN

Eccleston C, Baoru Y, Tahvonen R, Kallio H, Rimbach GH, Minihane AM. Effects of an antioxidant-rich juice (sea buckthorn) on risk factors for coronary heart disease in humans. *J Nutr Biochem*. 2002 Jun;13(6):346–354.

Yang B, Bonfigli A, Pagani V, et al. Effects of oral supplementation and topical application of supercritical CO2 extracted sea buckthorn oil on skin ageing of female subjects. *Journal of Applied Cosmetology*. 2009 Jan;27(1):13.

Yang B, Erkkola R. Sea buckthorn oils, mucous membranes and Sjögren's syndrome with special reference to latest studies. *Seabuckthorn (Hippophae L.): a multipurpose wonder plant. 3rd vol*. Delhi: Daya Publishing House. 2008:254–267.

Yang B, Kalimo KO, Mattila LM, et al. Effects of dietary supplementation with sea buckthorn (Hippophaë rhamnoides) seed and pulp oils on atopic dermatitis. *J Nutr Biochem*. 1999 Nov;10(11):622–630.

SILICA

A double-blind, placebo-controlled randomized study of the effect of Trica-Sil on several biochemical markers of the bone remodeling. *CERN* (Lorient, France) 2005. Corporate study.

Bremont JF. Pre- and post-treatment with Trica-Sil in dental implant patients: a review of 37 cases. Dental office (Nantes, France) 2007. Implantologist reports.

Davenward S, et al. Silicon-rich mineral water as a non-invasive test of the 'aluminum hypothesis' in Alzheimer's disease. *J Alzheimers Dis*. 2013;33(2):423–430.

In vitro evaluation of the effect of Trica-Sil on the metabolism of bone matrix. *Biopredic* (Rennes, France) 1999. Corporate study.

Jugdaohsingh H, Tucker KL, Qiao N, Cupples LA, Kiel DP, Power JJ. Dietary silicon intake is positively associated with bone mineral density in men and premenopausal women of the Framingham Offspring cohort. *J Bone Miner Res*. 2004 Feb;19(2):297–307.

Jugdaohsingh H. Silicon and bone health. *J Nutr Health Aging*. 2007 Mar-Apr;11(2):99–110.

Maya S, Prakash T, Madhu KD, Goli D. Multifaceted effects of aluminium in neurodegenerative diseases: A review. *Biomed Pharamcother*. 2016 Oct;83:746–754.

Rondeau V, Jacqmin-Gadda H, Commenges D, Helmer C, Dartiques JF. Aluminum and silica in drinking water and the risk of Alzheim'ers disease or cognitive decline: findings from 15-year follow-up of the PAQUID cohort. *Am J Epidemiol*. 2009 Feb 15;169(4):489–496.

Wang X, Schroder HC, Wiens M, Ushijima H, Muller WE. Bio-silica and bio-polyphosphate: applications in biomedicine (bone formation). *Curr Opin Biotechnol*. 2012 Aug;23(4):570–578.

ST. JOHN'S WORT

Fava M, Alpert J, Nierenberg AA, et al. A Double-blind, randomized trial of St John's wort, fluoxetine, and placebo in major depressive disorder. *J Clin Psychopharmacol*. 2005 Oct;25(5):441–447.

Linde K, Berner MM, Kriston L. St John's wort for major depression. *Cochrane Database Syst Rev*. 2008 Oct 8;(4):CD000448.

Linde K. St. John's wort—an overview. *Forsch Komplementmed*. 2009 Jun;16(3):146–155.

Schrader E. Equivalence of St John's wort extract (Ze 117) and fluoxetine: a randomized, controlled study in mild-moderate depression. *Int Clin Psychopharmacol*. 2000 Mar;15(2):61–68.

Singer A, Schmidt M, Hauke W, Stade K. Duration of response after treatment of mild to moderate depression with *Hypericum* extract STW 3-VI, citalopram and placebo: a reanalysis of data from a controlled clinical trial. *Phytomedicine*. 2011 Jun 15;18(8–9):739–742.

WHITE WILLOW BARK

Chrubasik S, Künzel O, Model A, Conradt C, Black A. Treatment of low back pain with a herbal or synthetic anti-rheumatic: a randomized controlled study. White willow bark extract for low back pain. *Rheumatology* (Oxford). 2001 Dec;40(12):1388–393.

Gagnier JJ, van Tulder MW, Berman B, Bombardier C. Herbal medicine for low back pain: a Cochrane review. *Spine* (Phila Pa 1976). 2007 Jan 1;32(1):82–92.

Schmid B, Lüdtke R, Selbmann HK, et al. Efficacy and tolerability of a standardized white willow bark extract in patients with osteoarthritis: randomized placebo-controlled, double blind clinical trial. *Phytother Res*. 2001 Jun;15(4):344–350.

DIET FOR A LONG LIFE

"Adult Obesity Facts." Centers for Disease Control and Prevention. Available at: www.cdc.gov/obesity/data/adult.html. Accessed: March 1, 2017.

"Adult Obesity Prevalence Maps." Centers for Disease Control and Prevention. Available at: https://www.cdc.gov/obesity/data/prevalence-maps.html. Accessed: March 1, 2017.

Chiuve SE, Rimm EB, Manson JE, et al. Intake of total trans, trans-18:1, and trans-18:2 fatty acids and risk of sudden cardiac death in women. *Am Heart J*. 2009;158:761

Clarke R, Lewington S. Trans fatty acids and coronary heart disease. *BMJ*. 2006 Jul 29;333(7561):214.

Mozaffarian D, Katan MB, Ascherio A, Stampfer MJ, Willett WC. Trans Fatty Acids and Cardiovascular Disease. *N Engl J Med*. 2006;354:1601

Steinberg D. Thematic review series: the pathogenesis of atherosclerosis. An interpretive history of the cholesterol controversy: part I. *J Lipid Res*. 2004 Sep;45(9):1583–93.

LOVE YOUR EXERCISE

Burgomaster KA, Howarth KR, Phillips SM, et al. Similar metabolic adaptations during exercise after low volume sprint interval and traditional endurance training in humans. *J Physiol*. 2008;586, 151–160.

Little JP, Safdar A, Wilkin GP, Tarnopolsky MA, Gibala MJ. A practical model of low-volume high-intensity interval training induces mitochondrial biogenesis in human skeletal muscle: potential mechanisms. *J Physiol*. 2010 Mar 15;588(Pt 6):1011–1022.

Perry CG, Heigenhauser GJ, Bonen A, Spriet LL. High-intensity aerobic interval training increases fat and carbohydrate metabolic capacities in human skeletal muscle. *Appl Physiol Nutr Metab*. 2008 Dec;33(6):1112–123.

Rakobowchuk M, Tanguay S, Burgomaster KA, Howarth KR, Gibala MJ, MacDonald MJ. Sprint interval and traditional endurance training induce similar improvements in peripheral arterial stiffness and flow-mediated dilation in healthy humans. *Am J Physiol Regul Integr Comp Physiol*. 2008; 295, R236–R242.

Tremblay A, Simoneau JA, Bouchard C. Impact of exercise intensity on body fatness and skeletal muscle metabolism. *Metabolism*.1994 Jul;43(7):814–818.

Index